MORE PRAISE FOR
THE NEW EDITION OF
THE COMPLETE BOOK
OF BREASTFEEDING

"I RECOMMEND THE BOOK TO ALL MY LAMAZE CHILDBIRTH CLASSES, AND ONLY WISH IT HAD BEEN AROUND WHEN I WAS BREASTFEEDING MY CHILDREN."—Barbara Silver, R.N., *APSO/Lamaze, ACCE*

"AN INVALUABLE HELP FOR CONTEMPORARY WOMEN—AND THE CHAPTERS ON WORKING MOTHERS AND SEXUALITY ARE SIMPLY SUPERB."— Barbara Seaman, Women's Health Activist, author of *The Doctors' Case Against the Pill*

"I READ THIS TRULY COMPLETE GUIDE WHEN I WAS EIGHT MONTHS PREGNANT, AND FOUND IT ENOR-MOUSLY HELPFUL AND INFORMATIVE."—Lonnie Bar-bach, Ph.D. Clinical Social Psychologist, author of *For Yourself: the Fulfillment of Female Sexuality*

"THE SECTION ON WORKING MOTHERS IS A MAR-VEL! THEY ESPECIALLY NEED THE UNIQUE BOND-ING THAT BREASTFEEDING OFFERS, AND THIS BOOK TELLS THEM EVERYTHING THEY NEED TO KNOW."—Reikie Ehrlich-Alles, President, *Long Island ASPO/ Lamaze*

"AN HONEST, UP-TO-DATE, REASSURING BOOK . . . CHOCK-FULL OF VALUABLE, PRACTICAL INFORMA-TION THAT IS JUST NOT TAUGHT IN MEDICAL SCHOOL."—Richard L. Saphir, M.D., Associate Clinical Professor of Pediatrics, Mount Sinai School of Medicine

"I HAVE REFERRED PARENTS TO THIS BOOK FOR MANY YEARS. THE NEWLY REVISED EDITION IS EX-CEPTIONAL IN EVERY WAY!"—Rosemary J. Diulio, R.N., Ed.M., Director, Parent Education, Maternity Center Associa-tion, New York City

ABOUT THE AUTHORS

Marvin S. Eiger, M.D., is a nationally known pediatrician and breastfeeding authority and is a strong advocate of the natural way—over half the babies in his care are breastfed. Educated at Harvard University, Dr. Eiger received his medical training at New York University School of Medicine and served his residency in pediatrics at Bellevue Hospital. A Fellow of the American Academy of Pediatrics, Dr. Eiger is presently Director of the Comprehensive Lactations Program at the Beth Israel Medical Center and is an Associate Clinical Professor of Pediatrics at the Mount Sinai School of Medicine.

Sally Wendkos Olds is an award-winning author of nine books and over 200 articles that have appeared in major national magazines. She nursed her own three daughters and wrote her very first magazine article about breastfeeding when her oldest child was an infant. Her textbooks on human development have been read by over one million college students, and her most recent book is THE ETERNAL GARDEN: SEASONS OF OUR SEXUALITY. She lives on Long Island with her husband.

TOTALLY REVISED

The Complete Book of
BREASTFEEDING

by Marvin S. Eiger, M.D.
& Sally Wendkos Olds

Photography by Roe Di Bona
Illustrations by Wendy Wray

BANTAM BOOKS
TORONTO • NEW YORK • LONDON • SYDNEY • AUCKLAND

To our children
from whom we learned so much

Nancy and Dorri Olds
Jennifer Olds Moebus
Michael and Pamela Eiger

This low-priced Bantam Book
has been completely reset in a type face
designed for easy reading, and was printed
from new plates. It contains the complete
text of the original hard-cover edition.
NOT ONE WORD HAS BEEN OMITTED.

THE COMPLETE BOOK OF BREASTFEEDING, REVISED EDITION

A Bantam Book / published by arrangement with
Workman Publishing Company, Inc.

PRINTING HISTORY
Workman edition published April 1972

Bantam edition / September 1972

Workman revised edition / January 1987

Bantam revised edition / October 1987

Book photographs: Roe Di Bona.
Book illustrations: Wendy Wray.

ISBN 0-553-26232-7

Published simultaneously in the United States and Canada

PRINTED IN THE UNITED STATES OF AMERICA

O   0 9 8 7 6 5 4 3

ACKNOWLEDGMENTS

We want to express our grateful appreciation to the many friends and colleagues who generously gave of their expertise and time, who contributed the fruits of their research, and who offered valuable suggestions to aid us in making this edition of our book as helpful as possible to nursing mothers. We owe a special debt to the following persons, who reviewed parts or all of the manuscript for the new edition and whose evaluations and suggestions were enormously helpful: Kathleen Auerbach, Ph.D., Jimmie Lynne Avery, Christopher R. Fletcher, M.D., Helen Rosengren Freedman, Frank R. Greer, M.D., Charlotte Lee-Carrihill, Toni Littlejohn, Jennifer Moebus, Frank A. Oski, M.D., Judith Palsgraf, R.N., Judith Roepke, R.D., Ph.D., Richard Saphir, M.D., Concepcion G. Sia, M.D., Barbara Silver, R.N., Christopher Springman, Frances Stout, M.S., R.D., Frank W. Summers, M.D., Maurice Teitel, M.D., Edith Tibbetts, M.Ed., Marian Tompson, Reginald C. Tsang, M.D., Elaine S. Turner, M.D., and Eleanor R. Williams, Ph.D., Jan Yager, Ph.D.

Our thanks also go to those whose research and thinking helped us shape the first edition, especially Harry Bakwin, M.D., Saul Blatman, M.D., T. Berry Brazelton, M.D., Michael J. Brennan, M.D., Nathaniel S. Cooper, D.D.S., Mary Cossman, Lois Dwyer, Paul Elber, Sylvia Feldman, Ph.D., Samuel J. Fomon, M.D., Florence Fralin, Vincent Freda, M.D., Lawrence M. Gartner, M.D., Barbara Goodheart, Elizabeth Hormann, Derrick B. Jelliffe, M.D., Tobe Joffe, Alice Ladas, Ed.P., Philip Lipsitz, M.D., Michael Newton, M.D., Niles Newton, Ph.D., Kathleen O'Regan, R.N., Alice Rossi, Ph.D., Asoka Roy, R.N., C.N.M., M.S., Benjamin Segal, M.D., Samuel Stone, M.D., Evelyn B. Thoman, Ph.D., Tilla Vahanian, Ed.D., the staffs of the departments of pediatrics at Beth Israel Hospital Medical Center and New York University Medical Center and of the Newborn Service at University Hospital, and, of course, the many mothers and fathers who shared with us their thoughts and feelings about breast-feeding.

We received valuable information and help from the following organizations and agencies: The American Academy of Pediatrics, The American College of Obstetricians and Gynecologists, The American Dental Association, The American Public Health Association, The American Medical Association, La Leche League International, International Childbirth Education Association, The Human Lactation Center Ltd., The National Institute of Child Health and Human Development, The New York Academy of Medicine, The American Cancer Society, Maternity Center Association, The Port Washington Public Library, and Health Education Associates, Inc.

We also want to express our gratitude to our publishers, Workman Publishing Company and Bantam Books, and especially to Peter Workman, Suzanne Rafer, Patty Romanowski, and Toni Burbank. Right from the start, through the life of the first edition and into this new edition, we have received the kind of enthusiastic support that nurtures and strengthens both books and authors.

And our very special thanks to Yaa and Kofi Brinkley, Jane, Ron, and Peter Brown, Katharine, Benjamin, and Joshua Zalusky, Craig and Dalva Senna, Natalie Weinstein, Lori, Eric, and Samuel Baumel, Amy Manso and Kira Manso Brown, Dolores DeLuise, Ariel and Carl Pellman, Bobbi Lurie, Ari and Michael Aster, Margaret, Tom, and Julia Preston.

Marvin S. Eiger, M.D.
New York, New York

Sally Wendkos Olds
Port Washington, New York

PREFACE

If you were living at some other time or in some other place, you might not need this book. You might even wonder about its purpose, since you would be getting much of the information in these pages from your mother, your aunts, your older sisters, and your neighbors. They would share with you their breastfeeding experiences and those of their mothers before them. As you saw them suckling their infants, you would pick up the "tricks of the trade" without even realizing it. It would never occur to you that you would not nurse your baby, because every baby that you had ever seen would have been fed at his mother's breast—except in the extremely rare case when a mother was too ill to nurse.

The paragraph you have just read appeared in the introduction to the original edition of this book, published in 1972. It is one of the very few paragraphs that have been carried over intact into this edition, for much has changed in the decade and a half since *The Complete Book of Breastfeeding* was first conceived. The year 1971 (when the first edition was being researched and written) marked the lowest rate of breastfeeding in the history of this country, when only one out of four women breastfed their newborn babies. Today, well over half of all American mothers nurse their infants, and among well-educated middle-class women, the incidence is even higher.

In the past fifteen years we, the authors (a pediatrician with a large number of breastfed babies in his practice and a medical writer who nursed her own three children), have seen an explosion of research into the properties of breast milk, the value of nursing for both mothers and babies, and the practices that enhance or hinder the course of breastfeeding. We have applauded professional organizations like the American Academy of Pediatrics, the Canadian Paediatric Society, and the World Health Organization as they issued strong statements urging mothers to nurse and urging medical professionals to help nursing mothers and their babies. We've been happy to note that today's physicians learn more about breastfeeding in medical school and are less likely to believe that formula is "just as good" as breast milk, and to see that more hospitals are instituting policies that promote breastfeeding rather than interfering with it.

Today, then, if you have questions about breastfeeding, you're more likely to have sources to go to—the doctors, nurses, and midwives who help you in childbirth, the friends and neighbors who are nursing or have nursed their own children, and a wealth of published material. Still, depending on where you live and where you have your baby, the information you get may or may not be helpful. In too many places you're likely to hear outdated, incorrect advice. Some medical professionals have not kept up with new research findings that invalidate what they learned in medical or nursing school. Some laypersons, especially those from a generation more familiar with bottle-fed babies, are still convinced of the myths and superstitions they heard in a less enlightened time.

Breastfeeding is easy; there is nothing complicated about it. Still, it is a skill that has to be learned, and it is an activity whose success depends on information and support. Nursing a baby may fulfill an instinctual drive, but both mothers and babies need to learn the actual procedures for breastfeeding and need to be reassured while they're learning. Some mothers intuitively know what to do, puzzled by no questions and troubled by no problems. Most new mothers, however, have questions about all aspects of infant care. Sometimes their lack of information about breastfeeding makes them hesitate to embark upon an adventure that seems strange and bewildering. Other times, they reluctantly switch to the bottle when, had their questions been answered and their problems solved, they would have preferred to continue being part of a nursing couple.

To help you do what you want to do and to make the most of what may be among the most memorable and enjoyable experiences of your life, we have updated and completely revised this book. It now includes findings from the most current scientific research as well as advice from nursing mothers themselves. It also addresses a number of lifestyle issues that are increasingly important to contemporary mothers. Thus you'll see more in this new, revised edition about diet and fitness, about breastfeeding for the working mother (including the best ways to express or pump and store breast milk), about breastfeeding as a sexual passage in the life of the mother, about nursing in public, and about nursing in a variety of special situations.

The three essential tools for successful breastfeeding are the knowledge of what to do, the confidence that you're doing the right thing for your baby and yourself, and the determination to persist in the face of any minor setbacks that may come your way. As authors who've learned much more about our subject since we wrote our first book, we hope that this new edition will help you develop all three of these tools

Marvin S. Eiger, M.D.
Sally Wendkos Olds

A Note about Language

Since babies come in two sexes, we write about them accordingly, alternating gender pronouns throughout the text. This seems to be the fairest solution to a problem that plagues most writers sensitive to the bias implicit in the English language.

We made another linguistic decision when we decided to refer throughout the book to "your husband" or "your baby's father." It's likely that most readers of this book are married, but also that some are not. If you're living with another adult, you can substitute his or her name in those places where we refer to a husband or to the baby's father. If you're raising your child alone, you may not be able to get the kind of help we suggest, but you can still, of course, breastfeed your baby and benefit from most of the suggestions in these pages.

Contents

4

Before the Baby Comes

5

The Care and Feeding of the Nursing Mother

10

11

12

1

Will You or Won't You?

Only in relatively recent times has there been any question as to whether or not a baby should be breastfed. In earlier days, if a mother was either unable or unwilling to nurse her baby herself, she had to find another woman to do it. Early in the twentieth century, however, the advent of dependable refrigeration and pasteurization and the development of ways to modify cow's milk for infant consumption meant that babies could be fed a specially formulated product that was both digestible and nutritious.

Today you have a choice in the way you feed your baby. You can decide whether you want to feed your baby with the milk produced by your own body the way mothers have done from time immemorial—or whether you want to take advantage of modern technology and provide your baby's nourishment in a bottle. Many factors will enter into your decision—the customs of your community; the attitudes of your doctor, your husband, your friends, and family; your lifestyle, including your work commitments; your personality; your feelings about mothering; and the degree of emotional support you receive.

In the United States, the nursing mother was for years the nonconformist, a member of a minority group. By 1971, formula feeding had become the norm in this country, with only one in four women nursing. Since then, however, the long-term trend away from breastfeeding has been reversed, so that today more than 60 percent of new mothers nurse their babies. Before you decide what you will do, you'll want to consider the advantages of breastfeeding and how it will fit into your personal situation.

You probably have heard many of the reasons why breast-feeding is good for babies, most of which we'll talk about in this chapter. You may not be as aware of all the benefits it can hold for you. One of the prime advantages for you is the all-around good feeling you're likely to derive from the experience.

THE ENJOYMENT FACTOR

Many women decide to breastfeed because they don't want to rob themselves of this rich experience, of the emotional satisfaction and enormous sense of fulfillment that nursing a baby can bring. As one mother told us, "There is something very right about a system that makes one human being so happy about being responsible for another. I could never have the same good feeling of accomplishment by relying on the neighborhood store or the dairy for my baby's milk. Knowing that I was giving him something no one else could give him created a tie between us that became one of my deepest joys."

In talking about their breastfeeding experiences, women often emphasize how good it feels (or felt)—emotionally, physically, and intellectually. One proof of the enjoyment many women get from this aspect of mothering can be seen in the fact that when a woman has breastfed one baby successfully, she almost always nurses the next.

Women who have bottle-fed one baby and nursed another tend to feel closer to their nursing infants in the early months of life. A common reaction is reflected in this statement from one such mother: "I never knew what I was missing by not nursing my first baby. I loved him and I enjoyed him, yes, but I never got so many of the little 'extras' that I get from this one—that little hand that touches my skin as she's nursing, the way she'll pull away from the breast, smile at me and go

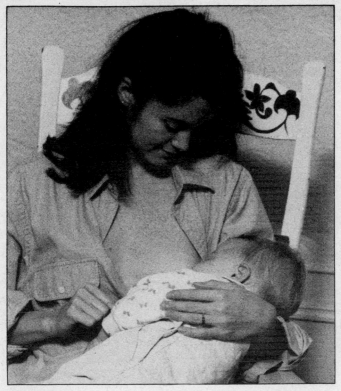

A loving moment shared by a nursing mother and her baby.

right back again, the happiness that I feel at being able to give her what she wants."

The "nursing couple"—mother and baby—forge an especially close and interdependent relationship. The baby depends upon the mother for sustenance and comfort, and the mother looks forward to feeding times to gain a pleasurable sense of closeness with her infant. If a feeding time is too long delayed, both members become distressed—the baby because of hunger and the mother because of uncomfortably full breasts. Each member needs the other, yearns for the other, is intimate with the other in a very special way. Because of this unique symbiotic relationship, many women consider the period of nursing among the most fulfilling times of their lives.

In addition, nursing can be an intensely pleasurable, sensuous activity, since suckling a baby gives rise to some of the same physical responses that occur in sexual activity, as we'll see when we talk about female sexuality in Chapter 10. And finally, knowing all the health benefits that breastfeeding confers on both mother and baby affirms a woman's conviction that she is making the best possible decision for herself and her baby. Let's see what some of these benefits are.

BENEFITS FOR THE BABY

Nutrition

Human breast milk is the ideal food for human infants. For the first four to six months, it is the only food a baby needs. Even after other foods are introduced into the baby's diet, breast milk continues to supply important nutrients such as essential fatty acids for proper digestion, and lactose for the proper growth of brain cells and the correct balance of amino acids (the building blocks of protein).

In recent years nutritionists have voiced concern about the overly high levels of protein in the American diet. Since cow's milk contains about twice as much protein as human milk, formula-fed babies usually receive more protein than they need. This protein overload may ultimately lead to problems with the baby's metabolism.

In the United States today, there's a new awareness of the serious problem of overnutrition; bottle-fed babies tend to be fatter than breastfed babies. One reason for this may stem from the fact that bottle-feeding mothers who see milk left in the bottle tend to encourage their babies to drain the last drop, while breastfeeding mothers usually assume that when their babies stop sucking, they've had enough.

Another way in which nursing may discourage overfeeding lies in the difference between the high-protein milk produced at the beginning of a feeding (fore milk), and the high-fat milk produced at the end (hind milk). The richness of the hind milk may make the baby feel full and send a signal that mealtime is over.

Health

Breast milk confers many other important health benefits. In underdeveloped tropical countries, the survival rate for the breastfed baby may be six times greater than for his bottle-fed cousin. And even among the children of middle- or upper-class parents in well-developed countries, breastfed babies are healthier.

•Breastfed babies make fewer visits to doctors' offices and hospitals than bottle-fed babies do, especially for diarrhea, other gastrointestinal disorders, rashes, and respiratory infections. They are protected in varying degrees from a number of other illnesses, including pneumonia, bronchitis, botulism poisoning, hyperthyroidism, influenza, polio, staphylococcal and other infections, including painful middle-ear infections.

•Breastfeeding may confer protection against rubella (German measles); it may also help to prevent breast cancer and heart disease in later life.

How does breastfeeding give this protection? In several ways, including the following:

•Mother's milk transmits antibodies and other protective substances to the baby. Eighty percent of the cells in breast milk are *macrophages*, cells that kill bacteria, fungi, and viruses; they also help to stop the growth of cancer cells.

•Scientists just discovered that a substance in human milk is so powerful that a solution with only a three-percent content of human milk killed half a culture of intestinal parasites in a test tube within 30 minutes, and a one-percent solution killed half in an hour; cow's or goat's milk would be unable to produce a similar effect.

•A factor in breast milk encourages the production of the baby's own antibodies.

•Other elements in breast milk also confer protection, as we'll see in Chapter 3, which contains a comparison of human milk with cow's milk.

•Some of the benefits of breastfeeding are procedural: Milk in the mother's breast cannot be contaminated by the harmful bacteria that can multiply in animal milk left out of the refrigerator for too long a period of time. It's always served in a clean container. It can't be overdiluted to save money. Mistakes can't be made in its preparation (as they are from time to time in baby formulas, sometimes with disastrous results).

In highly developed countries such as ours, where sanitary conditions are generally good, the gap in health between the breastfed and the bottle-fed baby is narrowed considerably. In addition, modern medical techniques can now vanquish many of the illnesses that used to be fatal to infants. Still, it's better to prevent disease than to cure it. And there's a great deal of evidence that breast milk does indeed have preventive, protective powers.

Digestibility

Babies can digest human milk more easily than the milk of other animals, probably because human milk contains an enzyme that aids in this process. Breast milk forms softer curds in the infant's stomach than cow's milk (the basis for most formulas) and is more quickly assimilated into the body system. While it contains less protein than does cow's milk, virtually all the protein in breast milk is available to the baby. By contrast, about half the protein in cow's milk passes through the baby's body as a waste product. Similarly, iron and zinc are absorbed better by breastfed babies.

Breastfed babies are less apt to get diarrhea, and they hardly ever become constipated, since breast milk cannot solidify in the intestinal tract to form hard stools. (When constipation does occur, a slight modification of the mother's diet can solve the problem.) While a breastfed baby may soil all of her diapers in the early days or go several days without a bowel movement later on, neither of these situations indicates intestinal upset. Some premature infants and other babies with sensitive digestive systems thrive only on breast milk. If their own mothers cannot or do not provide it, they may be able to get it from a milk bank.

A few such human milk banks exist around the country. Usually they're affiliated with hospitals, but some are independent. Most are small, charge little or nothing, and depend on the voluntary contributions of milk by other nursing mothers. Priority for milk is usually given to premature babies, babies who cannot tolerate formula, and babies who need fresh milk to fight infection. Information about such banks is available from breastfeeding support groups like La Leche League and International Childbirth Education Association. (For addresses and telephone numbers, see Chapter 4.)

Human Milk for Human Babies

The milk of every species differs in its composition from every other milk. We can logically assume that each animal produces in its milk those elements most important for the survival of its young. Human milk contains at least 100 ingredients that are not in cow's milk, and while artificial formulas can try to imitate mother's milk, it can never be duplicated exactly.

For one thing, breast milk changes in composition from day to day. For another, each mother's milk is custom-designed for her own baby: Women develop specific antibodies against the proteins in the food they eat themselves and against bacteria in their lungs and intestines. Thus, they manufacture the mix of antibodies best for their own babies. In addition, we're constantly discovering new ingredients in mother's milk. The perfect match between a baby and its mother's milk is dramatically evident in the case of premature infants: The milk of a woman who has delivered prematurely is higher in fat than that produced by the mother of a full-term baby and is, therefore, better suited to the needs of her preterm baby.

Through trial and error, formula manufacturers have learned which ingredients are essential for babies' nutrition. A few years ago when one manufacturer lowered the salt content in its formula, the resulting compound ended up with such a low level of chloride that babies who drank it became severely ill. An earlier fiasco had followed another manufacturer's move to use higher temperatures for sterilization; this destroyed vitamin B_6, an element that until then had not been known to be vital. Who knows what other ingredients will be identified in mother's milk for formula-makers to try to imitate?

Breastfed babies differ in many respects from their bottle-fed counterparts. The ratio of vitamins in their systems is different, as is the composition of various substances in their blood. The bacteria in their intestinal tract are strikingly different, consisting largely of *Lactobacillus bifidus,* a beneficial organism that prevents the growth of certain harmful bacteria and that's present in only small numbers in the stool of bottle-fed babies. *Lysozyme,* another substance found only in the stools of breastfed infants, also protects against harmful micro-organisms.

Breastfed babies even grow differently from bottle babies, who not only grow longer and fatter, but also develop bigger and heavier bones during the first year of life, probably due to the large amounts of calcium present in cow's milk. Formula-fed babies may grow faster than nature intended them to, showing an artificial growth pattern much like the Strasbourg geese that are force-fed to make them grow fat. Bigger is not necessarily better.

Teleology, the ultimate purpose or design in nature, is revealed in another way. Newborn babies see best at a distance of between 12 and 15 inches, precisely the distance of a baby's eyes from the face of a nursing mother. As Aristotle said so many centuries ago, "There is reason behind everything in nature."

Even though we don't know the precise reasons for, or the significance of, all the differences between the baby nourished at the breast and the baby fed from a bottle, it seems logical to assume that the best first food for your baby is the kind you provide yourself. As Dr. Paul György, the pioneering researcher who discovered vitamin B_6, said more than 60 years ago, "Human milk is for the human infant; cow's milk is for the calf."

Less Chance of Allergic Reactions

While many babies do well on formulas, occasionally an allergic reaction, such as indigestion or diarrhea, occurs. The mother faced with this problem may feel like a chemist in the lab as, on the advice of her doctor, she tries different proportions and different kinds of milks and sugars.

The breastfeeding mother never has this concern, since no baby is allergic to breast milk. Some babies do, however, develop allergic reactions such as vomiting, diarrhea, skin rashes, hives, or sniffles, to something in the mother's diet that's transmitted through the milk. As explained in Chapter 5, it's usually possible for the mother to identify and stop eating the allergenic food for the duration of nursing.

Some research suggests that breastfeeding reduces the likelihood of allergic reactions such as eczema, asthma, and runny noses. If true, this makes nursing a particularly compelling option in families with a history of allergies. Such families need to be alert to the possibility of cow's milk allergy, which is fairly common. Babies are usually protected from this as long as they're taking nothing but breast milk, and it seems that the earlier a baby with this predisposition receives cow's milk, the greater the risk of developing such an allergy.

Tooth and Jaw Development

Suckling at the breast is good for a baby's tooth and jaw development. Babies at the breast have to use as much as 60 times more energy to get food than do those drinking from a bottle. The nursling has to mouth much or all of the areola (the darker area around the nipple), move his jaws back and forth, and squeeze hard with his gums to extract the milk. To accomplish this arduous task, your baby has been endowed with jaw muscles three times stronger than yours in relation to body size. As these muscles are strenuously exercised in suckling, their constant pulling encourages the growth of well-formed jaws and straight, healthy teeth.

One factor accounting for many dental malformations that eventually send children to the orthodontist or the speech therapist is an abnormal swallowing pattern, known as "tongue thrust." This is very common among bottle-fed babies, but almost nonexistent among the breastfed. To understand why, we have to examine the mechanisms of feeding. The baby at the breast moves the lower jaw back and forth quite vigorously to stimulate the flow of milk, and then pushes the tongue upward against the flattened nipple to keep it in the mouth. As the milk begins to come, it is sucked in and swallowed. The entire process is then repeated, so that a feeding session involves a constant succession of chewing and suckling motions.

Bottle-fed babies don't have to exercise their jaws so energetically, since light suckling alone produces a rapid flow of milk. In fact, since milk usually flows so freely from the bottle,

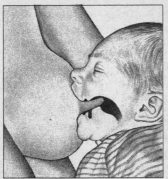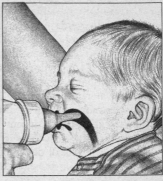

The baby at the breast pushes his tongue upward to nurse; the one at the bottle pushes his forward.

the baby actually has to learn how to protect himself from an oversupply so that he won't choke. He pushes his tongue forward against the nipple holes to stem the flow to a level that he can easily handle. The tongue that should be pressing upward has instead come forward, and a swallowing pattern that will most likely persist throughout life has begun. Many dentists believe that such a forward tongue thrust can result in mouth breathing, lip biting, gum disease, and a generally unattractive appearance.

The condition of "nursing bottle mouth" is much more common among bottle-fed babies. Letting babies fall asleep with a bottle of milk, juice, or other sweetened liquid can cause tooth decay in a pattern that corresponds to the area where the liquid comes out of the bottle. This pattern of decay is very rare among breastfed babies.

Another factor contributes to breastfed infants' healthy tooth and jaw development. Since they get more of the sucking that most babies seem to need, they're less likely to suck their thumbs. Bottle-fed babies have to stop sucking on the nipple as soon as the bottle is empty to avoid taking in air; your baby at the breast can continue in this blissful pastime until he or you decide he's been at the well long enough.

Of course, not all bottle-fed babies develop dental problems, and some breastfed babies do. In addition, new "orthodontic" nipples (the Nuk and the Kip) have been designed to avoid the development of "tongue thrust" and its inherent problems. Despite their much closer approximation to the human nipple, however, there's no doubt that the real thing will continue to remain superior to all its imitators.

The Natural Way

At a time when so much of our life has an unsettlingly unnatural aspect—with chemicals in the air we breathe, in the clothes we wear, and in the foods we eat—more and more of us

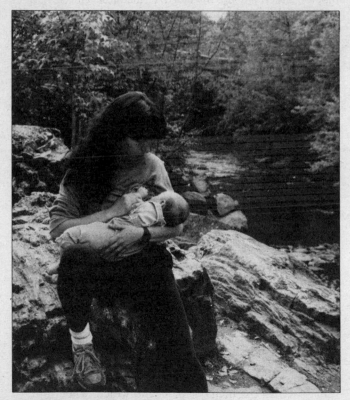

*Miles away from store or refrigerator,
a nursing mother can still feed her baby.*

are striving to recapture some of the natural joys of life on earth. When you breastfeed your baby, you know you're giving her the natural food intended just for her. Its purity is tainted by no synthetic compounds, no preservatives, no artificial ingredients. Breast milk is the ultimate health food.

If you're concerned about the environment your baby will grow up in, you can appreciate the ecological superiority of breastfeeding. Feeding the bottle-fed baby entails the use and disposal of innumerable cans and bottles of formula, the cardboard cartons that package them, and the baby's bottles and nipples, which are also discarded, either after one use or after a few months. Then there's the energy used to heat the milk, and the soap or detergents and water used to wash all that equipment.

Availability

Another advantage the nursling enjoys is the constant availability of milk. Her dinner is always ready, always at the right temperature, always at the right consistency. She doesn't have to struggle to get milk from a nipple with scanty holes nor does she have to gulp furiously to keep up with a gush from extra-large ones. No snowstorm, no flood, no car breakdown, no milk-driver's strike can keep her food from her. You don't have to worry about running short when you're out with your baby. As long as mother is near, so is sustenance.

Emotional Gratification

Much has been written and said about the psychological benefits that babies derive from breastfeeding. Dr. Niles Newton, a psychologist who has made extensive studies of lactation in humans and in laboratory animals, has found many psychological differences between breast and artificial feeding, most of which tip the scales in favor of nursing. For example, lactating mice demonstrate a greater drive than non-nursing mice in overcoming obstacles to reach their infants, indicating some mechanism in lactation itself that triggers maternal behavior. It may well be the hormone prolactin, which, when injected into a chicken will make her take care of nearby chicks, even if they aren't her own. Infants do seem to become attached to their mothers very early, as shown by the fact that one-week-old babies turn their heads more often and are more likely to suck toward breast pads that their own mothers had worn, compared to pads worn by other nursing women.

As a result of studies conducted over the past 50 years in order to correlate methods of infant feeding with later personality development, researchers have concluded that as important as early feeding experiences may be to a child's later development, there are so many variables in parent-child relationships that it's impossible to claim definitively that breastfeeding of itself is a prescription for healthy adjustment. The mother who reluctantly breastfeeds only out of duty communicates her resentment to her child. The mother who weans suddenly and traumatically can undo much of the good that's been built up in the nursing relationship. Breastfeeding, then, is not always psychologically superior to bottle feeding.

However, psychiatrists and other students of human and animal nature do state categorically that babies gain a sense of security from the warmth and closeness of the mother's body.

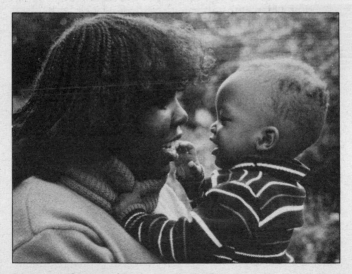

Sometimes playing with someone who holds you lovingly is just as much fun as nursing.

Also, it seems that the more intimate interaction between the breastfeeding mother and child, the warm skin-to-skin contact, and the more immediate satisfaction of the nursing baby's hunger would augur healthier psychological development. When you breastfeed your baby, you cannot be tempted—even on your busiest days—to lay your baby down with a propped bottle. You *have* to draw her close to you for every single feeding. While bottle-feeding mothers can also show their love for their babies by holding and cuddling them at feeding times, in actual practice they tend to do less of this. And while they *can* hold their babies next to their bare skin when they offer the bottle to simulate the body contact of nursing, they rarely do so. Research has proved the value of the sense of touch in many different settings. This basic element of breastfeeding is one of the most gratifying aspects of the experience, to both mother and baby.

Babies also gain a sense of well-being from secure handling, and nursing mothers often seem more confident. Whether the woman who's sure of her maternal abilities is more likely to breastfeed—or whether the experience of being a good provider infuses her with self-confidence—is hard to answer. Nursing mothers do seem more likely to know how to soothe their babies when they're upset, maybe because the very act of putting them to the breast is such a comfort that it isn't necessary to search for other means of reassurance. The breast is more than a pipeline for getting food into the baby. It's warmth; it's reassurance; it's comfort.

BENEFITS FOR THE MOTHER

Your primary reason for wanting to breastfeed is probably your awareness that it will be better for your baby. You may not have realized that nursing offers a world of benefits for you, too.

Good for Your Figure

Nursing your baby will help you to regain your figure more quickly, since the process of lactation causes the uterus (which has increased during pregnancy to about 20 times its normal size) to shrink more quickly to its prepregnancy size. During the early days of nursing, you can feel the uterus contracting while your baby suckles. As he nurses, he stimulates certain nerves in the nipples that bring about uterine contractions. These contractions hasten the uterus's return to its former size, while helping to expel excess tissue and blood. The uterus of the nonlactating mother always remains somewhat larger than it was before she became pregnant. Furthermore, since nursing uses up so many calories, you may be able to lose weight while eating more.

Contrary to popular belief, nursing does not break down the tissues in the breasts. Any changes in the breasts that occur, such as a loss of firmness, are the results of pregnancy, weight gain, heredity, and maturity, not lactation.

Convenience

Even today, when formula comes ready-mixed in nursing bottles, nursing is easier. In the area of infant feeding, no efficiency expert has been able to outdo nature. Your baby's daily batch of food prepares itself in its own permanent containers. It's so easy just to wake up in the morning, pick up the baby, and put her to your breast.

If you're using the kind of formula you prepare yourself, the difference, of course, is even greater. You don't have to mix formulas. You don't have to scrub and sterilize bottles and nipples. In either case, you don't have to go into the kitchen to heat up a bottle. You never have to make up an extra bottle at the last minute or throw out formula that your baby doesn't want. Working on the time-honored principle of supply and demand, your mammary glands produce the amount of milk your baby wants.

You'll find it easier to go visiting or traveling with your baby, since you won't have to take along bottles, nipples, and formulas, nor will you have to worry about refrigeration and dish-washing facilities. When you have to be separated from your baby (if you work, for example), you can express and store your milk or you can nurse when you're with your baby and offer formula when you're apart.

Your Health

Every new mother needs adequate rest. The many physiological changes of pregnancy, the hard work of labor and delivery, and the demanding care of a new baby all deplete your energy. When you breastfeed, you're able to relax during your baby's feeding times, since you cannot prop a bottle or turn the baby over to someone else while you run around doing chores.

An important health advantage is the likelihood that as a lactating woman, you won't resume menstruating as soon—not until six to 12 months after childbirth, compared to one and a half months afterward for the typical non-nursing mother. This is the only time in your reproductive life when you're not losing iron through the menses or through nourishing a baby in the womb. Thus, this is a chance to build up your stores of iron and correct any anemic tendencies you may have.

Economy

Breastfeeding saves money. If you eat properly, you don't have to change your diet. You just need to eat small amounts of extra food to make up for the calories you expend in producing and giving milk. This will cost you less than you'd have to pay for bottles, nipples, sterilizing equipment, and formulas. In recent years public health professionals have been mounting special campaigns to educate and help women in low-income groups, so that they can reap the economic benefits of breastfeeding.

Esthetics

If you have a sensitive nose you'll appreciate the fact that your breastfed baby smells better. Both bowel movements and excess milk spit up after feedings smell mild and inoffensive, unlike the strong odors of the bottle-fed baby.

Birth Control

Breastfeeding acts as a natural—although admittedly unreliable—means of spacing children. While your baby is receiving nothing but breast milk—no solid foods or formula at all—and is still being nursed at night, you're less likely to become pregnant than the non-nursing or partially nursing mother. This is because the fully lactating woman rarely ovulates. *Nursing a baby is not a guarantee against pregnancy, however.* While you are less likely to conceive while you're nursing, it's possible that you might become pregnant. *If you want to plan the size and spacing of your family, you need to use some form of contraception.* (See the discussion in Chapter 10 regarding birth control suitable for nursing women.)

WHY SOME WOMEN DECIDE AGAINST BREASTFEEDING

The reasons why women decide not to breastfeed are almost as varied as the arguments in its favor. There are very, very few instances when a woman cannot nurse her baby—when the mother has had surgery or trauma to the breasts that has severed the ducts, when she has a hormonal or glandular insufficiency, when she is so ill that she can't be with her baby, or when the baby has some condition making it impossible to nurse. Fortunately, such cases are extremely rare. Virtually every healthy woman can breastfeed her baby if she wants to.

Why do some women prefer not to? This question has no simple answer. Women say they don't want to breastfeed because:

•they're embarrassed about the idea;

•they're modest and neither want to nurse publicly nor have to run into another room whenever people are around;

•they think body secretions of any kind are "icky";

•they don't want to be tied down;

•they have to go back to work and don't want to start something they can't finish;

•their husbands don't want them to;

•they don't want to ruin their figures;

•they think they don't have the right kind of breasts;

•they're too nervous;

•they won't know whether their baby is getting enough to eat;

•the whole business just seems too complicated.

None of these reasons exists in a vacuum. Most were born in history, either society's or the individual's. Many stem from a lack of knowledge. While it's up to each individual woman to look at her own personal reasons for her choice, we can take a look at some relevant societal trends, and in the next chapter we'll answer some of the questions that are most often on women's minds.

How Our Society Has Influenced Women

At the beginning of the twentieth century, psychologists, psychiatrists, and physicians were convinced that babies developed best if they were raised according to certain hard-and-fast rules. Mothers were ordered not to feed—or even pick up—their babies more often than every four hours, no matter how piercing or pathetic the infants' wails. Bottle feeding was far better adapted to these practices. For breastfeeding requires flexibility, not rigidity; understanding of a baby's needs, not the ability to tell time; and an intuitive reaction, nor an adherence to a cultural fad. Also, because the child-care experts insisted that only they knew what was best for children, mothers believed them—and lost confidence in their own capabilities. Lack of confidence itself can sabotage breastfeeding.

At the same time these mothers were being intimidated in the nursery, they were asserting themselves on the street. Demonstrating to achieve the right to vote, smoking cigarettes in public, bobbing their hair, and daring to carve out their own careers, women were eager to free themselves from their traditional roles in the house. The baby bottle became an instant symbol of emancipation.

Furthermore, as the quality of formulas improved during the 1930s, the act of giving a bottle achieved a certain status of its own. Women who wanted to be modern wanted to bottle-feed. Unfortunately, this urge to keep up, to be "modern," has wooed many poor women in both developed and underdeveloped countries around the world away from the breast, often with disastrous results. When money is scarce, mothers dilute the milk and babies starve; when refrigeration and sanitation are inadequate, the milk becomes contaminated and the babies sicken. The World Health Organization, many individual governments, and a number of private health organizations have mounted major campaigns to encourage women to go back to safe, healthy breastfeeding.

Meanwhile, the modern counterparts of those feminists who moved away from breastfeeding—the well-educated, middle- and upper-class women who set trends—are now among its staunchest supporters. They have often, in fact, had to call upon the same qualities of strength and assertiveness to achieve their right to nurse as to achieve choice in other areas of their lives.

During the flapper era, tight binders hid and flattened women's breasts; by the 1940s, pin-up photos were gracing barracks walls, exhibiting the new ideal of feminine beauty—a pretty young woman with large breasts. These organs, molded into fashionably pointed shapes by the brassieres of the day, became purely decorative in nature, valued for their sexiness and forgotten for their functionalism.

More recently, as the braless look has become more widely accepted in society, as nudity has become more prevalent in the media, as the breasts have become somewhat de-emphasized as sexual symbols (often now taking second place to the derriere, the current star of ads for blue jeans), many women have become more comfortable with the notion of touching and baring their breasts, as least to the extent required for nursing. As we'll see in Chapter 8, it's also possible to nurse so discreetly that observers can't even tell what you're doing, which sets to rest a concern of many women and men.

Today's woman is more comfortable with her body than in times past, is concerned with fitness and health for herself and for her family, and is not embarrassed to be herself. Our ideals of beauty have changed from the heavily made-up, elaborately coiffed look of yesterday to a healthy, natural look. Thus, the contemporary woman is more likely to want to feed her baby in the way that seems the healthiest and the most natural.

These changes in society, along with new scientific research affirming the value of human milk, have contributed to the resurgence of breastfeeding. Probably the first half of this century in America will go down in history as an aberration in its temporary rejection of this age-old natural way of nurturing babies.

Still, even if you want to breastfeed, you may have many questions and concerns. Even after your questions are answered, you may decide that breastfeeding is not for you. You don't have to breastfeed to be a good mother. You shouldn't do something you find abhorrent to please your husband, your doctor, your mother, or your best friend. If you do, you're doomed to failure. How you feel about your children is more important than how you feed them. In one recent study, psychologists from Harvard University followed up 78 people in their thirties whose mothers had been interviewed 25 years earlier. These researchers found that the fact or the duration of breastfeeding, like many other specific child-rearing practices, had no discernible effect on the way these people turned out as adults. The only thing that did matter was whether the parents had truly loved their children—and had shown their children that love.

A baby raised in a loving home can grow up to be healthy and psychologically secure no matter how he receives his nourishment. While nursing is usually a beautiful, happy experience for both mother and child, the woman who nurses grudgingly, tight-lipped, and stiff-armed, because she feels she *should*, will probably do more harm to her baby by communicating her feelings of resentment and unhappiness than she would if she were a relaxed, loving, bottle-feeding mother.

WHAT WILL YOU DO?

We urge you to give breastfeeding a try. You might look on it as a thirty-day guarantee or your money back. Suppose you begin to nurse your baby and you decide that it's not for you. You haven't lost anything; you haven't invested in anything; you can always stop. The stores will always have those bottles, nipples, sterilizers, and formulas. You haven't made a lifelong commitment. You can change your mind.

On the other hand, if you decide to bottle-feed right away, it's much harder to change your mind later on. Initiating breastfeeding even after a week has gone by requires a great deal of determination, persistence, and patience. It has been done by mothers who found that their babies needed breast milk to survive and by women who discovered that bottle-feeding has its own problems, but it is not easy.

If you never give breastfeeding a chance, you may well look back on this time in later years and wonder whether you and your baby missed out on one of life's greatest gifts—the bond shared by the nursing couple. The regrets we have in life are less often for the things we have done than for those missed opportunities that will never come again. This priceless chance to nurse your baby comes only once in each baby's lifetime. Make the most of it. You may count these nursing days among the most beautiful and fulfilling of your entire life.

2

Questions That May Be on Your Mind

While most of the questions in this chapter are answered in some way elsewhere in this book, we're listing them here because they represent the most common concerns of women who are thinking about breastfeeding.

Q: Does nursing ruin the breasts?

A: No, it does not. Some women notice little or no change in their breasts even after bearing and nursing several children; others develop a definite droop after only one. The breasts of most women become less firm and less erect after childbirth, but these changes are caused by pregnancy, not by lactation. The extent of the change is determined by heredity, age, and partly by the amount of weight gained during pregnancy.

The breasts are larger during lactation, but usually return to their former size after weaning. Some women feel their breasts are smaller after nursing, some feel they are larger, but most experience no change at all. In any case, the die is cast by the time your first child is born; whether you nurse this child or not will have no permanent effect on the size and shape of your breasts. (The temporary effects are often wel-

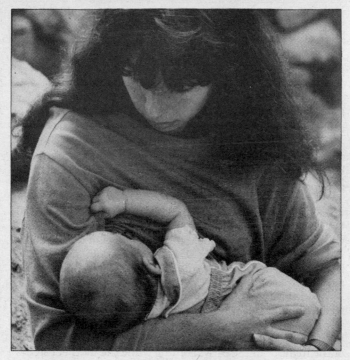

No one but this baby can see her mother's breasts, and onlookers may not even realize that she is nursing.

comed by small-breasted women. With the help of a support-ive bra and flattering clothing, fuller-bosomed women can feel and look good during this time.)

Q: Does nursing make a woman fat?

A: No, it does not. Many women have breastfed several chil-dren and ended up just as slim as they were before they became pregnant. Proper diet during pregnancy and lactation, com-bined with moderate exercise, will keep you slender. In fact, there's some evidence that nursing helps women to regain their figures, since the fat stores developed during pregnancy are laid down specifically for lactation. Women who do not nurse may have a harder time working off this fat.

Q: Does a nursing mother have to stay with her baby 24 hours a day? I can't bear the thought of being so tied down.

A: Nursing a baby does restrict your freedom somewhat—just as parenthood itself is restrictive. You can, however, work out a schedule so that you have a great deal of liberty once your milk supply is established and your baby has developed more regular feeding times. Many working mothers breastfeed despite full-time schedules. (For suggestions, see Chapter 9.)

Many women leave a bottle for the baby before leaving for an occasional afternoon or evening out. The bottle can contain formula or your own milk. Advice on these feedings is given in the Appendix.

The first couple of months after childbirth tend to be confining for most mothers, no matter how they feed. You'll need to rest and you'll want to stay near your baby, both of which will keep you close to home. So even if you plan to go back to work or to resume an active schedule that would make breastfeeding difficult, you can still nurse your baby in the early months.

A few women successfully combine breast- and bottle-feeding on a regular basis. The babies of working women usually receive one or more bottles while their mothers are on the job. Some fathers feed their babies bottled milk in the middle of the night or in the early morning while the mother catches up on sleep. And some mothers of twins regularly alternate breast and bottle for each baby.

The course of breastfeeding almost always runs smoother when the mother provides almost all of the baby's nourishment herself and relies on only an occasional bottle. In most cases it's safest to wait a while before combining the two forms of feeding, preferably after the mother's milk supply is well established—six to eight weeks after birth. But combining the two forms of feeding on a daily basis works well for some women, preventing that tied-down feeling.

Q: I like the idea of nursing, but won't it be embarrassing to have to expose my breasts to feed the baby?

A: Our society's erotic interest in women's breasts has generated a taboo against showing them in public, thus keeping many women from nursing. It's a shame that the nursing mother, one of the loveliest subjects in art or nature, should be such a rare sight in our society. If you had been more accustomed to seeing breastfeeding women, you probably would not be so shy about doing it yourself.

You can deal with these feelings in a number of ways, however. When you begin to nurse, insist on strict privacy. In the hospital ask the nurse to draw a screen around your bed; at home find a quiet nook where no one is likely to disturb you. Chances are that after you have nursed your baby a few times, you'll be so gratified by the experience that you won't find it embarrassing.

Furthermore, by wearing the right kinds of clothes, you can nurse in such public places as airplanes, department stores, or park benches without anyone being aware of what you're doing. Advice on nursing modestly in front of friends or even in front of delivery people who suddenly appear at the door is given in Chapter 8.

Q: I hear so many stories about women who really wanted to nurse their babies but had to switch to the bottle because for some reason they couldn't nurse. How can I be sure this won't happen to me?

A: It's true that in our country many women stop breastfeeding very early. Many others, however, continue to nurse for many months—or years. When encouragement, information, and support are available, more than 95 percent of all women can breastfeed. The first two weeks are the most crucial: It's important to build your support network, reach out for help, and have the attitude that you can overcome any problems that arise. With this viewpoint, you're virtually assured of a gratifying nursing experience.

Q: Does breastfeeding hurt?

A: Some women experience no discomfort at all, but most do feel some tenderness, usually in the very beginning as the baby starts to attach to the breasts. This initial soreness, apt to be felt most strongly by fair-skinned blondes and redheads, usually goes away in a few days. A number of simple measures to alleviate this discomfort are described in Chapter 7.

Q: What happens when the baby's teeth come in?

A: The baby who's nursing properly cannot bite the breast. Some teething babies may try to bite down toward the end of a feeding, after their initial hunger has been satisfied. As little as they are, these infants can and should learn not to do this. If you can anticipate when the biting is likely to start, take the baby off the breast ahead of time. Should he persist, say "No!" in a firm voice and take him off the breast immediately. After getting this reaction a couple of times, he'll learn not to bite.

Q: Why do some women have milk and not others?

A: Every healthy woman who has ever had a baby has had milk in her breasts. The functioning of the let-down reflex (explained in Chapter 3) may be somewhat inhibited in certain women in certain circumstances, but virtually every woman can get her milk to her baby.

Q: My mother didn't have enough milk to nurse me. Will I take after her?

A: The ability to breastfeed is not inherited. Virtually all cases of insufficient milk supplies are due to mismanagement of one sort or another and to lack of encouragement from doctors, hospitals, families, and friends. Your mother may not have had enough milk because at the time you were born, the value of breastfeeding was not appreciated. Today, with a renewed realization that this is the best way to feed an infant, we have relearned the old ways of building a mother's milk supply (explained in Chapters 7 and 8) and are constantly coming up with new ways to help mothers and babies.

Q: I'm almost perfectly flat-chested. How could my breasts possibly hold enough milk to nourish a baby?

A: The size of the breasts has no relation at all to their ability to produce milk. Size is determined by the amount of fatty tissue in the mammary glands. Since this fatty tissue is not at all involved in the process of making or ejecting milk, small breasts are not an obstacle to feeding a baby. Small-bosomed women breastfeed very successfully, and some even donate extra milk to milk banks for the benefit of sick or premature babies. See Chapter 3 for a detailed explanation of how the breasts make and give milk.

Q: How can I breastfeed if I have inverted nipples?

A: Many nipples that seem inverted (pushed in) work themselves out during pregnancy so that they're able to function normally after the baby is born. Sometimes exercise during pregnancy (like "nipple rolling") will help to bring out such nipples. Other cases are helped by wearing special breast cups. Nipples that don't respond to any of the measures described in Chapter 4 are extremely rare. Even in these cases, a baby may be able to grab hold of the areola and manage to get the milk despite the lack of a protractile nipple.

Q: How can I tell if my milk is rich enough for my baby?

A: If you are in reasonably good health and eating adequately, your milk will have enough of the essential elements that your baby needs. Don't worry about its bluish, watery appearance—that's what human milk is supposed to look like. See Chapter 5 for suggestions on the diet that you need.

Q: Suppose my milk doesn't agree with my baby?

A: Breast milk agrees with every baby. No baby is allergic to it. However, some babies do react to certain foods that you eat, and if you find that your baby is rejecting the breast or developing colicky symptoms, examine your diet for possible offenders, as explained in Chapter 5.

Q: I've always been the "nervous type" and I hear that you have to be calm to breastfeed. Am I doomed to failure?

A: It's true that a calm, relaxed mother usually has an easier time breastfeeding than does a tense, nervous one. And during times of emotional upset, the flow of milk may be considerably decreased due to an inhibition of the let-down reflex. The quality of the milk, though, is unchanged, and many women whose lives are very stressful nurse successfully. If you find it hard to relax when you start to nurse, there are a number of ways you can help yourself, as explained in Chapter 8.

For many women, the act of breastfeeding is a relaxer itself. This is probably due to the action of the hormone *prolactin*, which is released by the process of lactation, as explained in Chapter 3. Laboratory studies have shown that female rats fight less, maintain their body temperature better, and respond less to stressful situations when they're lactating. This moderation of the nursing mother's responses probably serves to protect babies from extreme changes in maternal behavior caused by outside stress. So you may be among the many "nervous types" who discover a new calmness through nursing.

Q: I want to breastfeed, but my husband doesn't like the idea. Is it worth making an issue about this?

A: Only you can decide how strongly your husband feels, how much of his opinion is based on lack of knowledge (which you can help to correct), and whether you should take a stand. The help and reassurance of a supportive husband are enormously valuable, so it pays for you to make an extra effort to find out what his objections are and to address them as well as you can. He may need both information and reassurance. It may also help to point out some of the advantages nursing holds for him (like relieving him of the responsibility for those middle-of-the-night feedings). Many a husband initially opposed to his wife's breastfeeding has become one of her staunchest supporters.

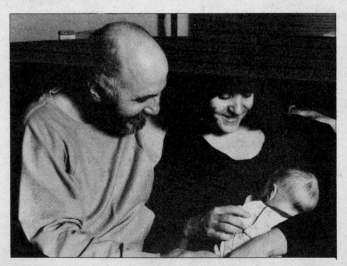

Many men become strong supporters of breastfeeding when they learn how it benefits the whole family.

Q: Ever since I decided to breastfeed, everyone has been trying to talk me out of it. How can I deal with all this opposition?

A: Opposition to breastfeeding is less common these days than it was a few years ago, but women still sometimes hear put-downs like, "You wouldn't make a good cow," "Why can't you be like everyone else and do the natural thing—give the baby a bottle?" "What are you trying to prove?" or "What? You're *still* nursing?" Or they're discouraged in more subtle ways by people who blame every little upset on the milk (or what they diagnose as your lack of it), or by doctors who suggest that you stop breastfeeding whenever you run into a minor problem.

When these situations arise, try to understand why people say these things and respond accordingly. When people have good intentions but poor information about the normal course of breastfeeding, you can enlighten them. When a trace of jealousy affects a grandmother (when she sees that you don't need her help) or a friend (who had an unsatisfactory nursing experience), you can help build up *their* morale. And when a doctor seems to be misinterpreting your questions, thinking that you're asking for permission to stop nursing, while you're actually asking for support and information, you can make an effort to be clearer in your communication.

In any case, once you make your decision to breastfeed, stick with it. You may not be able to change other people's minds, but you don't have to let them change yours, either.

Q: How will my older children react?

A: They'll respond to your own attitude. If you let them know that you're doing the right thing, they'll accept this. If you feel guilty and afraid of making them jealous, they'll sense your vulnerability and will capitalize on it. One recent study found that the older siblings of babies who were bottlefed misbehaved more at feeding time than did the siblings of babies being breastfed. Apparently, then, breastfeeding doesn't seem to add to the older children's stress.

Many women especially appreciate the opportunity to breastfeed a second child. As one mother said, "There are so many more distractions in my life now that I welcome the nice, quiet time that nursing affords, and I find I nurse this baby oftener than I did my first." For more about emphasizing the positive with the older brothers and sisters of a nursing baby, see Chapter 8.

Q: I am a single mother. Will it be too hard for me to take on the responsibilities of breastfeeding?

A: If you are the only parent in the home because you are separated or divorced from your husband, because you have been widowed, or because you have never married, you can still breastfeed. In fact, some single nursing mothers find that they especially appreciate the activity of nursing itself, partly because it ensures them of close physical contact with another human being and partly because of the often relaxing properties of the high levels of prolactin in their system. Your life is apt to be difficult in many ways because you don't have a partner to help you share the responsibilities of child care. You may be overwhelmed by the feeling that you have too much to do and too little time and energy to do it with.

It's particularly important, however, to take as good care of yourself as you can and to make special efforts to locate people who can become part of your support network. This is one time in your life when you don't want to become too isolated. You may find help from an organization of other divorced women or widows, or from a breastfeeding group. Call upon your family and friends—anyone who can offer encouragement, as well as practical help. And try not to let your day-to-day practical concerns overshadow the pleasures you can get from this time in your life. It makes its demands on you, but it also proffers rich rewards.

Q: I hate milk. Do I have to drink a quart a day to make milk?

A: You don't even have to drink a cup a day. While milk is an excellent source of protein, minerals, and vitamins, it's not the only source. You can either substitute other foods or take a vitamin and mineral supplement.

Q: Do I have to eat special foods while I'm nursing?

A: That depends on what you've been eating up till now. If you've been eating a variety of healthful foods, you don't have to change your eating habits—except to take in about 500 to 600 extra calories a day to make up for the ones you use in making and giving milk. If your diet has been deficient, however, this is a good time to make a change. Suggestions for a well-balanced diet are given in Chapter 5.

Occasionally you may find that certain foods you eat may upset your baby's stomach; common offenders are cow's milk and gas-producing foods in the cabbage family. Or your baby may seem especially wakeful after you've been drinking a lot of coffee. You can then cut back on the foods in question while you're nursing. Some babies don't react to any foods.

Be sensible, though. One mother called her pediatrician to say that her baby was fussy and asked whether it might be due to the fact that she had eaten chocolate the night before. When the doctor asked her what she had eaten, she replied, "Half a cake." It's surprising she wasn't on the phone to her own doctor.

Q: Can I breastfeed if my baby is born by a cesarean section?

A: Yes, the milk comes in just as quickly after a surgical birth as it does after a vaginal delivery. You may not feel up to nursing as soon as you would otherwise, but as soon as the anesthetic wears off, you can start to nurse. You'll probably want to rest more at home, which will improve the quality of your milk supply. More about this in Chapter 7.

Q: Can I breastfeed while I'm menstruating? I've heard that milk given at this time isn't good for the baby.

A: You may not menstruate at all while you're nursing. If you do, there's no reason not to nurse during your period. You may find that the hormonal changes connected with the menstrual cycle may temporarily lessen your supply of milk. If this happens, nurse more frequently. In any case, only the quantity of milk will be affected—not the quality.

Q: Does breastfeeding prevent pregnancy?

A: The definitive answer to this question is "Sometimes." Large-scale surveys of nursing, partially nursing, and non-nursing mothers in many countries around the world give rise to the conclusion that "breastfeeding is nature's contraceptive." On a societal level, breastfeeding may be more important than contraception in limiting family size. The individual woman who wants to prevent pregnancy, however, cannot count on breastfeeding for birth control.

Generally, if your nursing baby is receiving no supplemental bottles or solid food and is being nursed during the night as well as during the day, the hormonal balance in your body will prevent ovulation and therefore pregnancy for three to six months or even longer. Generally, you will have one sterile menstrual period warning you that you are about to ovulate. But you can't depend on it. Women have become pregnant while fully lactating and before their menses have resumed. So if you want to plan the size and spacing of your family, you need to put your trust in some other method of contraception, as discussed in Chapter 10.

Q: If I do become pregnant, can I continue to nurse my first baby?

A: You can continue to breastfeed, although it's probable that your milk supply will diminish somewhat after the first few months of your pregnancy. While some women nurse one child right through pregnancy and then nurse both the first and the second, this can pose problems. Lactation and pregnancy both demand a certain amount of energy from the mother; the two of them together may take too much of a toll. Also, you need to be sure that the infant gets the colostrum she needs and an adequate supply of milk, which may be difficult if you're also nursing a toddler. (Colostrum is a fluid secreted by the breasts for the first few days after childbirth, which is especially rich in antibodies, proteins, and other elements.) Most women around the world wean a nursling as soon as they learn that they're pregnant.

Q: Can I breastfeed a premature baby who has to stay in the hospital for several weeks?

A: Many mothers give their milk to their premature babies by expressing it and taking it to the hospital every day until the babies can nurse at the breast. Recent research has found that the milk of women who have delivered prematurely has more fat than that of women who have had full-term babies. For this reason it's better for premature babies to get their own mothers' milk than to receive pooled milk from a milk bank.

Therefore, many women feel it's worth the effort to maintain their supply of milk until the baby comes home. More about this in Chapter 13 and in the Appendix.

Q: Can I still breastfeed after cosmetic surgery?

A: You may be able to, depending on the kind of surgery you had and when you had it. In recent years more surgeons have tried to perform breast operations in a way that would permit future breastfeeding. If you had augmentation surgery to make your breasts larger and if the implant does not come into contact with mammary tissue, you can probably breastfeed. If you had reduction surgery to make your breasts smaller and if the nipple/areola complex is still attached to the breast tissue beneath it, you can probably breastfeed. For more on this topic, see Chapter 13. You'll also want to consult your own surgeon.

Q: I've heard that environmental contaminants like the insecticides DDT, dioxin, and dieldrin, the PCBs (polychlorinated biphenyls), and other chemicals are in breast milk. How harmful are they to babies?

A: Many women have been alarmed by "scare" reports that imply that the presence of such chemical residues in mother's milk makes it dangerous for babies. The truth is that *there is absolutely no medical evidence that breastfed babies suffer any ill effects from such chemicals*—except for a few rare cases of heavy occupational or accidental contamination. Scientists who have studied the levels of such pollutants in milk have stated repeatedly that the advantages of breastfeeding far outweigh the risk of harm from these chemicals.

Human milk does contain these pollutants, as does the milk of every mammalian species that has been investigated. While some human milk does contain these chemicals at levels higher than that allowed in milk for commercial sale, this commercially acceptable rate is an extremely conservative one. It is an estimate that about one thousandth of the dose is needed to cause harm. Actually, no one knows the point at which such contaminants become dangerous.

Since DDT and PCBs have been banned or restricted for some years, the levels of these chemicals are declining. Citizens need to put continual pressure on governmental agencies to monitor the use of new chemicals that may be just as pervasive, and to study their effects on human beings.

Meanwhile, what should nursing mothers do? Under ordinary conditions it's not necessary to have your milk tested, even if you live in an area where these chemicals are at high levels. As pediatrician Dr. Edward Kendrick wrote in *Pediatrics*, the journal of the American Academy of Pediatrics, in 1980, "Neither the experts nor local physicians can decipher the results." The only time it might make sense to have your milk analyzed would be if you were exposed to a highly concentrated dose of chemicals, either through an accident, exposure at work, or massive ingestion of contaminated foods, and if you or your baby showed any symptoms of chemical poisoning. Fortunately, this kind of experience is extremely rare.

Pregnant and nursing women should, however, take these basic precautions:

•Do not eat freshwater fish from waters known to be contaminated. (For information about suspect waters and fish species, call your state's Department of Environmental Conservation.)

•Peel or thoroughly wash fruits and vegetables to get rid of pesticide residues.

•Cut away the fatty portions of meats, poultry, and fish, since chemicals tend to be concentrated in the fat.

•Avoid dairy products rich in butterfat.

•Do not go on a crash diet during pregnancy or lactation, since a sudden loss of weight mobilizes fat cells and releases contaminants into other parts of the body where they may reach the baby.

•Avoid using pesticides and stay away from places where they are used, but if you *must* use them, use the nonaerosol kind.

3

The Miracle of Lactation

This chapter deals with some of the medical and scientific aspects of breastfeeding: how the breasts make milk and get it to the baby, how lactation may postpone menstruation and pregnancy, and the chemical compositions for colostrum, breast milk, and cow's milk. You're likely to find the sections, "Changes in the Breasts after Childbirth," "The Let-down Reflex," and "Menstruation, Ovulation, and Pregnancy" particularly helpful in understanding how breastfeeding works and what is happening in your body. Some of the other material here is rather technical, and you may want to skim through this chapter and read only those parts that answer your questions or look back later as questions arise. If you read it all, we feel you'll agree that *lactation*, the process by which a mother feeds her newborn baby with the milk produced by her own body, is truly a miracle of biologic design.

BREAST DEVELOPMENT

To understand how the breasts develop and function, we have to know a little bit about our bodies' glandular systems. Those parts of the human body that develop secretions are called glands. The endocrine glands (*endo* means within) secrete hormones, powerful chemical substances that pass directly into the bloodstream and then travel to other parts of the body. These hormones influence such basic processes as growth, sexual development, and even the formation of personality. The exocrine glands (*exo* means outside) secrete substances into ducts that are carried through the body. The breasts are exocrine glands that are stimulated, both in their development and in their production of milk, by the hormones of the endocrine glands.

These *mammary glands*, as the breasts are medically termed, got their name from *mamma*, the Latin word for breast. (Most likely, the early Romans got this word from their babies who closely associated their mothers with their source of food and directed their first word to both.)

Your mammary glands began to develop when you were a six-week-old embryo in your own mother's womb; the main milk ducts in your breasts were already formed by the time you were born. Right after birth, your breasts may even have been swollen and excreted a small amount of milk, once known as "witch's milk." (This very common phenomenon among infants of both sexes, which subsides after a few days, is caused by the stimulation of the infant's mammary glands by the same hormones produced by the placenta to prepare the mother's breasts for lactation.) Your mammary glands were inactive from that time until shortly before the onset of puberty, when hormones began to flood your body.

Changes of Puberty

Your body then took its first step toward changing from that of a girl to a woman when your pituitary gland, the "master gland" of the endocrine system, sent a message to your female sex glands, the ovaries, directing them to make *estrogen* in sharply increased amounts. Estrogen is the principal female hormone, the substance responsible for the growth of female-patterned body hair; for the sexual maturation of the genital organs; and for the development of feminine contours, including the swelling of the breasts. The pituitary gland also stimulated the manufacture of other female hormones, most notably *progesterone*, a hormone that actively prepares the body for pregnancy.

A combination of growth hormones and female sex hormones spurred the development of your breasts throughout your adolescence, until you reached your full body growth sometime in your late teens or early twenties.

BREAST ANATOMY

Your breasts are delicate organs made up of four basic kinds of tissue: the *glands* that secrete milk, the *ducts* that carry it, the *connective tissue* that supports and attaches the breasts to the muscles of the chest, and the *fatty tissue* that encases and protects these other structures.

Just as women differ in height, general body build, and facial characteristics, they vary considerably with regard to the size and shape of their breasts; furthermore, most women have one breast that's larger than the other. Whether your breasts are broad or narrow, rounded or conical, high or sloping, small or large, you can still nurse your baby. The size of your breasts is determined by the amount of fatty tissue they contain. Since the only purpose of this tissue is to encase and protect the more functional elements, it has no bearing at all on your ability to produce and give milk. You can be an excellent breastfeeder, no matter what the size or shape of your breasts.

The Nipple

Let's look at the breasts with a baby's-eye view. The nipple is the handle by which the infant grabs hold of the breast, and also the spout through which she receives her milk. The size of the nipple is as unimportant for nursing as is the size of the breast itself. Each nipple, which may be cylindrical in one woman and conical in another, has 15 to 25 tiny openings through which milk is excreted. As the nursing baby stimulates the many nerve endings in the nipple, this causes uterine contractions that help return the uterus to its prepregnancy size. Due to the smooth muscle fibers of the nipple, it becomes firm and erect when stimulated by cold, by sexual excitation, or by tactile stimulation like the mouth movements of the nursing baby.

When the nipple becomes erect (from the baby's suckling

or from sexual excitation), it becomes smaller and firmer, and its muscle structure exerts pressure to empty the milk pools.

The nipples of some women are *inverted*, that is, flat or folded in. Sometimes by the end of pregnancy they protrude normally and come out fully when the baby starts to nurse. Occasionally, however, such nipples remain inverted and pose a problem to the baby who cannot grasp the breast. Fortunately, this condition is almost always correctable by the measures described in Chapter 4.

The Areola

Surrounding the nipple is a darker-colored circle called the *areola*, which in most women measures between one and two inches in diameter, but which can be considerably larger. During pregnancy, the *Montgomery's glands* in the areola become enlarged and resemble little pimples. They remain quite noticeable throughout pregnancy and lactation, when they secrete a substance that cleanses, lubricates, and protects the nipple during nursing. The antibacterial properties in this substance also help to prevent infection in both mother and baby. After lactation, these glands recede to their former unobtrusive state.

The areola and nipple are darker than the rest of the breast, ranging from a light pink in very fair-skinned women to a very dark brown in others. The areolar pigmentation deepens in pregnancy and remains darker during lactation, after which the color fades somewhat; it never reverts, however, to the lighter shade it was before pregnancy. The darker color of the areola may be some sort of visual signal to newborns, since they must close their mouths upon the areola, not upon the nipple alone, if they are to obtain milk.

The Milk-Making Apparatus

Directly beneath and behind the areola is a group of *milk pools*, upon which the suckling baby puts pressure. These pools, known scientifically as *lactiferous sinuses*, are widened parts of the *lactiferous ducts*, or milk-carrying canals, which transport the milk to the nipples.

There are from 15 to 25 ducts, each of which empties into

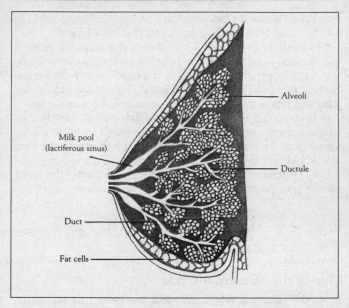

*A cross-section of the breast showing
how the milk gets to the baby.*

the nipple. The ducts branch off into smaller canals called
ductules within the breast. At the end of each ductule is a
grapelike cluster of tiny rounded sacs called *alveoli*, in which
the milk is made. Both the ducts and the alveoli are lined with
cells that contract so as to squeeze the milk into and through
the duct system. Each cluster of alveoli is referred to as a *lobule*
(a small rounded organ); a cluster of lobules is called a *lobe*.
The lobes, each of which is a miniature gland, are situated at
the base of the breast next to the chest. There are from 15 to
25 lobes in each breast, each lobe connected to one duct, each
duct emptying into one nipple opening.

The Supporting Structure

The breast is supported by the muscles attached to the ribs,
the collarbone, and the bones of the upper arm near the
shoulder. External support can also come from a well-fitting

bra. While wearing a bra or going without one has no effect at all upon the breastfeeding function, the force of gravity will tend to pull down the heavier breasts of the pregnant or nursing woman. A supportive bra helps to prevent undue stretching of the suspensory ligaments of the upper part of the breast. Some doctors feel that a woman whose breasts are wide at the base will retain her figure, whether or not she wears a bra.

In some cultures, women deliberately pull at their breasts to make them longer, so that it will be easier to nurse a baby strapped to their backs. Since this is probably not your aim, you would probably have the best chance for preserving your figure if you wear a good bra, even for sleep, during the latter part of your pregnancy as well as during lactation.

CHANGES IN THE BREASTS

During the Menstrual Cycle

From the time you reach the *menarche* (your first menstrual period) until you arrive at the menopause, a rhythmic cycle regulates your body. Every month your system produces a series of hormones that prepare your body to bear children, thickening the uterine lining and increasing the blood supply. In the months when you do not conceive, these preparations are washed away at the time of the menses. Ever optimistic, however, your body begins the entire cycle anew the next month.

The female sex hormones, estrogen and progesterone, produce changes in your breasts in the hope that this will be the month that sperm and egg will find each other to create a new being. Just before you menstruate, your breasts may enlarge and may feel tender as well. This is because the high levels of estrogen in your body make the blood vessels and gland ducts in the breasts increase in size somewhat during this premenstrual phase, in preparation for a possible pregnancy. (While the estrogen stimulates growth, it inhibits the production of milk. This is why your breasts will not begin to produce milk until after the birth of your baby and the delivery of the placenta.) Once menstruation begins, the breasts quickly return to their previous state. If, however, you become pregnant, the heightened levels of sex hormones in your body produce many changes in your breasts.

During Pregnancy

When you first go to have your pregnancy confirmed, your doctor will perform a pelvic examination and will closely examine your breasts for signs that you have indeed conceived. Some of these signs that appear by the fifth or sixth week of pregnancy include a persistent fullness and tenderness of the breasts similar to premenstrual sensations, the sudden prominence of the glands of Montgomery, and the enlargement and darkening of both the nipples and the areolae.

The complete duct system develops only now, when you are pregnant, and is completed sometime during the middle trimester (three-month period) of your pregnancy. At this point your breasts can secrete milk. Thus milk is available for your baby even if you should deliver prematurely.

By the time your baby is born, glandular tissue has almost completely replaced the fatty tissue in your breasts. The development of this glandular tissue is responsible for the enlargement of the breasts during pregnancy and lactation. By the time of your baby's birth, your breasts will be larger by about a pound and a half each.

The *placenta*, that organ that transmits nourishment and oxygen from your system to your unborn baby's, also has another function. It serves as a chemical factory that in early pregnancy takes over from your ovaries the job of producing large amounts of hormones. Somewhere around the fifth month of your pregnancy, the placenta begins to produce a new hormone, *human placental lactogen*, which stimulates the development of the alveoli, the milk sacs. Once these are formed, your breasts begin to produce "early milk," or *colostrum*, a sticky, colorless, or slightly yellowish liquid that may occasionally drip from your nipples during the latter part of your pregnancy. (More about this later.)

During pregnancy your body experiences rising levels of a hormone that's very important for lactation, *prolactin*. Your pituitary gland has been producing prolactin all your life, but its release is usually blocked by a recently discovered hormone in the brain known as a *prolactin-release inhibiting factor* (PIF).

During pregnancy prolactin levels are high, but its action is inhibited by the high levels of estrogen in your system.

After Childbirth

Once your baby has been born and the placenta has been delivered, the estrogen and progesterone levels in your body drop sharply. No longer inhibited by estrogens, your prolactin level rises sharply, enabling the full-scale production of milk within 24 to 48 hours after childbirth. Your baby's suckling stimulates the nerves that join the hypothalamus and the breast, thus limiting the secretion of PIF and permitting the production of more prolactin.

The changed hormonal balance in your body sets in motion a chain of events necessary for lactation to occur. Extra blood is pumped into the small blood vessels of the alveoli, causing these vessels to enlarge and to become visible beneath the skin, and making the breasts firmer and fuller. The manufacture of milk and the vascular expansion are responsible for the engorgement experienced by many—but not all—women. This *engorgement* (swelling caused by the pressure of the newly produced milk) and the temporary discomfort associated with it is almost always relieved by the baby's early and frequent nursing. (This is discussed in more detail in Chapter 7.)

The woman who does not breastfeed is apt to experience a great deal of discomfort from engorgement, which in her case may last from 24 to 36 hours. She may develop fever, headache, and throbbing pains in her breasts and under her arms. A firm bra and a mild pain reliever like aspirin usually help to relieve discomfort until her breasts stop producing milk. In the absence of a suckling baby, this should happen within a few days. While medication is often administered to a non-nursing mother to dry up her milk, the strongest factor in drying up the milk is the lack of stimulation to the breasts. If a baby does not nurse and if the milk is not otherwise removed from the breasts manually or with a pump, the alveoli get the message that they are not needed and they stop producing milk.

Immediately after birth, the cells in the center of the alveoli undergo fatty degeneration and are eliminated in the first milk as colostrum. At any point from as soon as 12 hours after birth to as late as four days afterward, the colostrum is replaced by the true milk. Generally, the sooner and more frequently the baby is put to the breast, the sooner the mother's milk comes in. The milk also comes in sooner for a woman who has previously nursed a baby, since the duct system in her breasts is already stretched and better able to transport the milk to the milk pools, where the baby can get to it.

THE LET-DOWN REFLEX— HOW THE BABY GETS THE MILK

The woman whose *let-down reflex* is operating well is usually overjoyed, not "let down" in the sense of feeling disappointed. This was originally a dairy term, referring to a cow's ability to let down her milk. Also known as the *milk-ejection reflex (MER)* and, in England, the "draught" (pronounced "draft"), the let-down gets the milk to the baby.

As your baby suckles, she stimulates the nerve endings in your nipples, which then send signals to your pituitary gland,

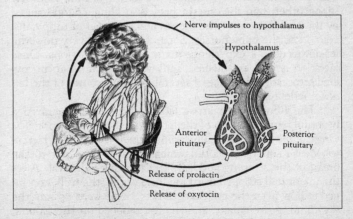

The baby's suckling initiates nerve impulses that direct the endocrine system to produce the hormones prolactin (which makes the milk) and oxytocin (which causes contractions that send the milk into the milk pools).

directing it to continue to produce the hormone prolactin. The prolactin signals the alveoli to produce milk. As long as your breasts are suckled, they will continue to make milk.

Your baby's suckling also causes your pituitary to release another important hormone, *oxytocin*. Oxytocin travels through the bloodstream to the breast, where it causes the little cells lining the alveoli to contract, thereby squeezing the milk from the alveoli into the ducts. As the milk enters the ducts, the cells along the walls of the ducts also contract, sending the milk out to the milk pools beneath the areolae. While prolactin makes the milk, oxytocin makes it available to the baby. (Recent animal research suggests that oxytocin also plays a part in the release of prolactin. This hormone also causes the uterus to contract during lactation, orgasm, and childbirth.)

In the early stage of lactation, it takes anywhere from several seconds to several minutes of the baby's suckling to produce a let-down reflex. After lactation is well established, you may find that hearing your baby cry or even just thinking about him will bring it on. Some signs of the let-down reflex are a tingling sensation in the breast, the dripping of milk before the baby starts to nurse, the release of milk from the nipple other than the one the baby is suckling, cramps caused by the contractions of the uterus, and the relief of nipple discomfort as the baby nurses. Some women with very powerful let-downs do not experience many of these sensations. Once lactation is well established, milk may spray from an uncovered breast for a distance of several feet at the onset of the let-down reflex.

The Renaissance artist Jacopo Tintoretto portrayed a beautiful representation of the let-down reflex in his work, *The Origin of the Milky Way*. The painting tells the story of Hercules, Zeus's son by a mortal woman, whom Zeus put to the breast of the sleeping goddess Hera to make immortal. After the infant had stopped drinking Hera's milk, the milk continued to flow from the goddess's breasts. Some went up into the sky, forming the galaxy, and the rest dropped on the ground, forming a garden of lilies. The British scientist S.J. Folley points out that this picture illustrates two important attributes of the milk-ejection reflex: first, that the stimulus of suckling creates an increased pressure of the milk inside the breasts, causing it to spurt from the nipples and secondly, that even though only one breast may be suckled, milk will flow from both.

In recent years, hormone preparations available in the form of a nasal spray or a tablet held in the mouth have been administered by some doctors to women whose let-down may be a bit slow in getting started. While this may be helpful to some nervous, high-strung women, many doctors feel that it is unnecessary and that any woman, if she gives herself time—sometimes up to several weeks—will develop an adequate let-down reflex.

The let-down reflex has a strong psychological base. The pituitary gland, which controls the release of oxytocin, is itself controlled by the hypothalamus. This walnut-size organ in the brain is often referred to as the "seat of emotion," since it receives messages about the individual's psychological state and, acting on these messages, sends its own orders to the glands, translating emotions into physiological reactions. The emotions, therefore, exert a powerful influence on such hormone-regulated functions as the menstrual cycle, childbirth, and lactation.

Some nursing failures can be attributed to a failure of the let-down reflex to function normally. Pain, embarrassment, or distraction can inhibit this reflex and hold your milk back from your baby. If your nipples hurt, your let-down may not work right. If you are distressed by the disparaging remarks of relatives and friends, your let-down may let you down. If you overtire yourself, don't eat properly, and don't respect your own needs for privacy and for relaxation, you may make the milk—but you may not be able to get it to your baby.

This is why it's important to prepare yourself for breast-feeding, both physically and emotionally. Chances are that even if you did nothing and knew nothing, you might still be blessed with good milk production and an active milk-ejection reflex. But the more you know and the better you can manage the course of breastfeeding, the better your experience will be.

MENSTRUATION, OVULATION, AND PREGNANCY

Women who do not breastfeed usually begin to menstruate and ovulate within one to three months after childbirth, while nursing mothers may not resume their cycles for more than a year. Your baby's suckling at your breast maintains high levels of prolactin in your system. The prolactin tends to suppress the action of your ovaries, preventing them from producing the hormones that trigger *ovulation*, the periodical release of *ova* (eggs). Most women do not ovulate or menstruate at all while their babies are receiving no food other than breast milk and are suckling frequently, day and night. If you are not releasing fertilizable eggs, you cannot become pregnant.

As soon as supplementary bottles or solid foods are added to the diet, the baby's sucking becomes less vigorous and the prolactin level in the mother's system drops. When the baby does not nurse for long stretches of time (during the night, or during the day for working mothers), prolactin levels also drop. When there is not enough prolactin to inhibit ovarian function, the mother again resumes her regular ovulatory and menstrual cycles.

There's a great deal of variability among women. One woman may have one "sterile" menstrual period before ovulation begins; that is, she may begin to menstruate but not yet be able to conceive. Another is fertile with her first menstrual period after childbirth. Some women don't begin to ovulate and menstruate for several months after their babies are completely weaned from the breast. Others ovulate even while they're fully lactating and before their menses resume. So while you're *less likely* to conceive when your baby is totally breastfed, you *might* become pregnant. Since it's impossible to tell when a particular woman will begin to ovulate, if you want to space your children you will want to use some kind of contraception. (Birth control for nursing mothers is discussed in Chapter 10.)

COLOSTRUM,
THE EARLY MILK

For the first one to five days after birth, your breasts secrete colostrum, the sticky clear or yellowish fluid that they have been producing since the latter part of your pregnancy. This is an ideal first food for your baby for several reasons. While it's similar to true milk, it's easier to digest and richer in disease-fighting antibodies. Its composition is different in other ways, too. It contains more protein, minerals, salt, vitamin A, and nitrogen. (Proportionately, it has nearly three times the amount of protein as mature milk, because it has several amino acids and antibody-containing proteins that are not found in mature milk.) It has higher levels of the antibody *secretory IgA* and higher numbers of white blood cells. It's lower in calories since it has lower levels of fat and sugar. The fat it does have is, however, higher in cholesterol.

The main function of colostrum seems to be to protect the newborn against infection, but it also may provide important nutrients. It has been shown to be especially beneficial for sick and premature infants. One important function it performs is a laxative one of cleaning out the *meconium* from the baby's bowels. This is greenish-black waste matter formed in the baby's intestinal tract before birth.

Over the past 20 years, more than 30 components have been identified in human colostrum, 13 of which are unique to breast milk. Some animals are known to receive immunity from certain diseases by drinking their mother's colostrum. Antibodies from colostrum have been found in the feces of breastfed babies, but not in those who receive only formula, and thus it seems quite possible that the breastfed baby's superior resistance to disease is in part due to these early antibodies. The value of the colostrum is a prime argument for feeding newborns as soon and as frequently as possible. It's also a good reason for beginning to breastfeed even if you feel you can do it for only a short time.

THE MILK

After the colostrum period has run its course, the true milk comes in. First, from about six days to two weeks after birth, the breasts secrete what's known as *transitional milk*, and then from two weeks on, they produce *mature milk*. What is this milk like?

Like the milk of other species, human milk is mostly water—88 percent. Its nutrient portion is made up mostly of fat (55 percent), then carbohydrates (37 percent), and finally proteins (8 percent). While this ratio is fairly constant, there is some variability from woman to woman and in the same woman at different times. Some of this variation stems from the mother's diet. The vitamins and minerals she gets will be reflected in her milk, as will the kind of fats she eats. As we'll see in Chapter 5, it's important for breastfeeding women to eat a variety of different kinds of foods. Aside from ensuring the healthiest balance of nutrients in the milk, a good diet will assure a greater volume of milk.

Milk composition varies during a single feeding session. The milk secreted at the beginning of a feeding, the *fore milk*, is leaner than the *hind milk* secreted toward the end of the feeding, which may be 50 percent higher in fat. The high-fat content of hind milk may give babies a feeling of fullness, letting them know that it's time to stop eating. Milk composition also seems to vary from one feeding to another, although research is somewhat conflicting on this. Some studies have shown it to be richest in fat in the morning, while others have shown it to be lean.

The protein content of milk also varies, with slight differences recorded even between the left and right breasts. Substantial change takes place over the course of nursing, as the very high protein level in the colostrum drops sharply in the first week and then gradually after that throughout lactation. After one year babies generally need other sources of protein.

The milk of every mammal has the same basic structure, but there are striking differences in chemical composition and proportion among the milks of various species. It seems reasonable to suppose that the milk of each species is especially suited to the needs of its young. The whale, for example, gives milk rich in fats and calories—elements important for survival in cold water. The milk of the rabbit is high in protein, which is important for the rapid growth of young rabbits. Even though we're constantly learning more about the unique structure of human milk, we'll probably never be able to identify every single one of its more than 100 different components. Over the last 20 years, hundreds of scientific papers have been published on the biochemical properties of human milk. The box on the following pages (Differences Between Cow's Milk and Human Milk) shows some of the differences between these two types of milk.

Aware of the differences between human milk and raw cow's milk, manufacturers of formula products use the latest scientific knowledge as a guideline for the preparation of nutritionally sound baby formulas. They use tables of recommended minimum daily requirements—and all their ingenuity. Most formulas, for example, replace the butterfat in cow's milk with some combination of oleo, soy oil, corn oil, coconut oil, palm oil, olive oil, or peanut oil. They experiment with various types of sugars, add substances to help the baby's body synthesize fatty acids, and in other ways try to copy breast milk.

From time to time, however, scientists discover new elements in breast milk, requiring modifications of cow's milk. One of the most exciting discoveries of recent years has been the finding that the composition of the milk secreted by women who have given birth prematurely is different from that of women who have borne a full-term baby. Nature's design is so elegant that each mother of a preterm baby produces milk that has the specific constituents needed by her own baby; it is higher in protein, fats, and the salts sodium and chloride. Thus it's better constituted to meet the needs of the tiny premature baby. It's most probable that, with all our scientific know-how, we'll never be able to isolate, identify, and copy all the ingredients of human milk—the best food for the human body.

Differences Between Cow's Milk and Human Milk

	COW'S MILK	HUMAN MILK
Color	Creamy white, due to high level of fats.	Bluish cast reflects lower fat content. Toward the end of a feeding, when fat content is higher, it looks creamier.
Vitamins	More D and K. Virtually no vitamin C.	More A and E, which may protect against anemia. Mother who eats well produces enough vitamin C for her baby. Babies need supplemental vitamin D if they don't get enough exposure to the sun and if their nursing mothers are strict vegetarians. Vitamin K should be administered to newborns to aid in blood clotting.
Iron	Very little.	Twice as much iron which is

		better absorbed by breastfed baby (probably because of the presence of *lactoferrin*, an iron-binding protein that is very abundant in human milk, barely present in cow's milk). Baby's iron requirements for first six months of life are met.
Other Minerals	Four times the amount of calcium, six times the phosphorus, and twice the sulphur as human milk. The bottle-fed baby excretes a large portion of these minerals as excess.	Zinc is more available in breast milk, preventing one skin disorder that's never seen in breastfed babies.
Protein	More than twice as much, in a form utilized less efficiently by the baby. (Current medical thinking is	Different kinds of proteins: Whey proteins (such as lactoferrin and secretory IgA) are abundant in human milk, while casein is the

(Continued on the following pages)

	COW'S MILK	HUMAN MILK
	that present recommendations for infant protein needs are based on cow's milk and may be set too high.)	prime protein in cow's milk.
Sugar	Half that in human milk.	The type in human milk may be responsible for the acidity of the breastfed baby's intestinal tract and the absence of many bacteria that cannot live in an acid environment.
Fats	Usually polyunsaturated vegetable fats are put into formulas to replace saturated fats in cow's milk.	High in saturated fats (and thus cholesterol), helps babies insulate nerves, form new cells, and maintain immunology. Breastfed babies have higher cholesterol levels, which may help

		them handle cholesterol better later in life. This may be why breastfed babies are apt to have lower cholesterol levels as adults. Human fat globules are smaller. Babies absorb human milk fat more efficiently than cow's milk fat.
Enzymes		Contains *lipase*, an enzyme that helps babies digest the milk.
Growth Modulators		Ingredients in human milk that help various cells develop and differentiate; these factors may have other roles, too. *Taurine*, an amino acid, aids in digestion and is also thought to be important in brain and nervous system development.

4

Before the Baby Comes

Long before you feel your baby's first stirrings inside your womb, you can prepare for breastfeeding. Getting information about what to expect during labor and delivery and early and thorough prenatal care will improve your chances for happy childbirth and breastfeeding experiences.

During the months before your baby's birth, you'll have a number of decisions to make. You'll need to decide what kind of medical and birth practitioners you want, where you want to have your baby, and what kind of delivery you want. You'll be taking a new look at your diet in these months and eating more and perhaps differently from the way you did before you became pregnant. (See Chapter 5 for suggestions on diet.) If you plan to go back to work soon after your baby's birth, you'll want to make inquiries and perhaps arrangements for child care. (See Chapter 9 for issues concerning breastfeeding for the working mother.)

CHOOSING YOUR HEALTH CARE PROVIDERS

Because the kind of medical and nursing care you and your baby receive before, during, and after the birth has such a far-reaching impact on your physical health, you want to be sure that the people you consult for help at these times are knowledgeable and skilled. Because the way you feel about the experiences of pregnancy, childbirth, and your family relationship has such a major influence on the emotional well-being of everyone in your family, you want to feel comfortable and happy with your helpers.

For More Help During Pregnancy

Since this book is mostly about what happens *after* your baby is born, we'll talk here about only a few of the issues you'll be dealing with ahead of time. For more detailed help you'll want to read material specifically oriented to the concerns of pregnancy. Two excellent books, which raise many questions and provide many helpful answers, are *What to Expect When You're Expecting* by Arlene Eisenberg, Heidi Eisenberg Murkoff, and Sandee Eisenberg Hathaway, R.N. (Workman, 1984) and *The Maternity Sourcebook* by Wendy and Matthew Lesko (Warner Books, 1984). For help with child-care choices and negotiating maternity leave, see *The Working Parents Survival Guide* by Sally Wendkos Olds (Bantam, 1986).

You have a number of choices at every stage of the reproductive process, as indicated in the thumbnail sketches in the box on page 58 (Types of Health Care Providers). The kind of practitioner you choose will depend on many factors—the community you live in, your philosophy about childbearing and medical care in general, your physical condition, your financial considerations, and possibly the personality of the particular practitioners you meet. You may want an older, well-established parent-figure type, or you might be happier with a partner-type close to your own age. You may have a gender preference. The location of the practitioner and the medical facility she or he is affiliated with may be important as well.

To help you decide, you can talk to friends, as well as representatives of childbirth education organizations. You can also consult books about pregnancy that describe these specialties in greater detail.

FINDING POSSIBLE CANDIDATES

To find the right person(s) for you—who are skilled, who share your philosophy about childbearing, and who are both knowledgeable and enthusiastic about breastfeeding—you can:

•ask friends who have recently had babies;

•ask your family doctor or gynecologist;

•call a local hospital or birthing center and ask them to recommend one or more people on their staff;

•call your local medical society and ask for recommendations;

•call representatives of the following organizations. Look in your local telephone directory first; if you don't find a listing, contact the national offices.

•ASPO/Lamaze (American Society for Psychoprophylaxis in Obstetrics, Inc.), 1840 Wilson Blvd., Suite 204, Arlington, VA 22201. (703-524-7802).

•ICEA (International Childbirth Education Association), P.O. Box 20048, Minneapolis, MN 55420–0048. (612-854-8660).

•La Leche League International, 9616 Minneapolis Ave., Franklin Park, IL 60131. (312-455-7730).

•American Academy of Family Physicians, 1740 W. 92nd St., Kansas City, MO 64114. (816-333-9700).

•International Lactation Consultant Association, P.O. Box 4031, University of Virginia Station, Charlottesville, VA 22903.

•American College of Obstetricians and Gynecologists, 600 Maryland Ave., S.W., Suite 300, Washington, DC 20024. (202-638-5577).

•American College of Nurse-Midwives, 1522 K St., N.W., Suite 1120, Washington, DC 20005. (202-347-5445).

•American Academy of Pediatrics, 141 Northwest Point Rd., Elk Grove Village, IL 60007. (800-433-9016).

•NAACOG (Nurses Association of the American College of Obstetricians and Gynecologists), 600 Maryland Ave., S.W., Suite 200 East, Washington, DC 20024–2589. (202-638-0026). (This organization of obstetric, gynecologic, and neonatal nurses conducts special programs for lactation consultants.)

•American Academy of Husband Coached Childbirth, P.O. Box 5224, Sherman Oaks, CA 91413. (818-788-6662).

Making Your Selection of Health Care Providers

Once you have the names of one or more practitioners in the categories you're looking for, you'll want to make your selection based on a number of criteria. Basically, you'll want to know the following:

•**Medical competence.** You can ask personnel at an accredited hospital or maternity center whether a practitioner is affiliated with the institution and has staff privileges (the ability to admit and treat patients), you can contact the appropriate organization to find out whether a practitioner is a member, or you can consult your library's copy of *The Directory of Medical Specialties* for information about a doctor's credentials. Or you can ask the receptionist or the practitioner about degrees and/or certification.

•**Fees.** Ask the receptionist or practitioner.

•**Breastfeeding knowledge and enthusiasm.** Ask the practitioner what percentage of his or her patients nurse their babies (the higher the percentage and the longer they nurse, the more helpful the practitioner is likely to be) and how available she or he is to answer questions outside of regular office visits.

•**Other issues.** To find out how a birth attendant feels about

Types of Health Care Providers

•*Obstetrician-Gynecologist:* Most women in America have their babies with the help of a physician who specializes in treating women and in delivering babies. Such a doctor will see you periodically throughout your pregnancy, will monitor the progress of your baby in the uterus, will deliver your baby, will examine you a few weeks after childbirth, and then will see you periodically throughout your life for routine checkups and care of your reproductive organs and your breasts. This doctor will not care for any other parts of your body or for any other members of your family.

•*Family Physician:* This up-to-date version of the general practitioner who takes care of everyone in the family is a far cry from the old-fashioned "GP" who used to make house calls in a horse and buggy. Family practice has been a recognized medical specialty since 1969, and family physicians can now receive certification after passing rigorous examinations enabling them to be the doctor of first contact. Family physicians can provide a continuity of medical care born from long years of treating family members. Some family doctors do not deliver babies, however. So you may have to turn to another practitioner for the birth, after which you can return to your familiar family doctor.

•*Nurse-Midwife:* These practitioners hold degrees in nursing and certification in midwifery, based on special experience and training designed to help them care for women with low-risk pregnancies and uncomplicated births. They work in conjunction with physicians in private practice, in maternity or birth centers, and in some hospitals. If complications arise they have back-up medical help. They are likely to devote more time to their patients than do medical doctors and to place more emphasis on emotional, as well as physical, support.

•*Lay Midwife:* The tradition of women who are not medically trained but who assist women in giving birth is an old one. Such practitioners, who usually learn from an apprenticeship, are legally permitted to practice in a few states. They espouse a natural philosophy in which they feel their role is not to intervene in the birth, but to provide emotional and perhaps spiritual support to the mother and to lend a pair of helping hands when she needs them. They also offer experience-based advice.

•*Pediatrician:* These physicians are specially trained and certified to take care of children from birth through adolescence, although some pediatricians continue to see their patients into young adulthood. Since they usually see at least one parent when they see a child, they come to know the entire family and often serve as the doctor of first resort for everyone. If you plan to consult a pediatrician for your children, it's a good idea to choose one at least three months before your due date. While this doctor will not care for the developing fetus, she will be able to examine your baby immediately after birth. If you deliver prematurely or if any complications arise with your baby's health, you'll feel more confident placing your baby's care in the hands of someone you have already met rather than having to deal with a complete stranger.

•*Lactation Consultant:* This is a new kind of health professional who has taken a special interest in breastfeeding and may have received special training, qualifying him or her to be an educator or consultant. A movement has begun to develop educational programs and certifying examinations for such consultants, who can then be available for telephone or in-person counseling for simple breastfeeding problems, either in private practice or in affiliation with a pediatrician, a hospital, or a maternity center. At present there is no universal certification requirement, programs vary considerably in their requirements, and some consultants are self-certified. As in the case of anyone you consult with regard to your or your family's health, it's important to check out qualifications.

the use of anesthesia, forceps, episiotomies, induction of labor, enemas, shaving, cesarean deliveries, breastfeeding immediately after delivery, and so forth, and how a doctor feels about circumcision, the initiation of solid foods, and other baby-oriented issues, you'll probably do best to raise these issues at your preliminary consultation. This is also a good time to ask about provisions for emergencies and back-up coverage in case you can't reach your own practitioner.

The Consultation

Call the practitioner's office and ask whether you can make an appointment for a consultation. If so, ask what the fee is, as compared to a complete examination. If not, go in for a complete examination. Ask your husband to go with you, since this decision will affect both him and his child, too.

Before you go, prepare a list of the questions you want to ask (with the most important ones first so you'll be sure to ask them). If you go in with a fair, nonbelligerent attitude, you should get a friendly and open-minded reception. If you don't—if the practitioner seems impatient or annoyed with your questions, wants to impose his or her views on you, or tries to soothe you with a "doctor-knows-best" attitude—you will have learned something valuable right at the beginning, and you may want to continue your search for a more compatible caregiver.

If you emerge from the consultation feeling confident that you made the right choice, your shopping is over. If you're not completely convinced, you don't have to say anything yet. Meet the other people on your list and then make up your mind.

You may find that you're not 100 percent happy with any of the practitioners you meet. Few matchings are perfect—most of us don't love everything about our spouses or our children, either. But if the good outweighs the bad by a comfortable margin, you're probably headed for a comfortable situation. Supportive health care providers are enormously helpful, but you can have a good nursing experience without them. You can find your own support among your family, your friends, and written materials. You can take the best that your practitioner has to offer—and help him or her learn through your experience—and both of you will gain.

As you read this, you may be well along in your pregnancy—and unhappy with your relationship with your practitioner. Or your baby may be born already and you feel that the doctor you've chosen is not as helpful as you had expected. Changing birth attendants or doctors is not a decision to be undertaken lightly, but it is possible. This is your pregnancy, your labor, your birth experience, and your baby. While the practitioner may be an expert in the field, you are an expert on your body and your own child. Your first obligation is to your own and your family's mental and physical health, not to your practitioner's feelings. Besides, health care professionals are made of pretty durable stuff; they recognize that they can't be all things to all people and that sometimes a switch is better for everyone concerned. The possibility of such a change is an important reason for not prepaying your entire obstetric fee.

CHOOSING WHERE YOU'LL GIVE BIRTH

At about the same time that you choose your birth attendant, you'll be deciding where you want to have your baby. The practitioner of your choice may not have staff privileges at the institution of your choice, so you may have to compromise. On the facility, there are three basic options:

•**Hospital.** While many hospitals are big and impersonal, with rigid rules that often seem designed for the smooth functioning of the institution rather than for the individual, others are run with the comfort of the patient more in mind. In recent years, as hospitals have competed more for fewer maternity cases, they have become more responsive to the desires of patients. Many now have rooming-in policies so that babies can stay in the mother's room for much or all of the day, permit fathers or other labor coaches to remain with the mother during labor and birth (including cesarean births), and offer such other aspects of family-centered maternity care as birthing rooms, family rooms that let siblings be present during childbirth, and queen-size beds that allow fathers to spend the night.

The Department of Health of New York State has mandated that all hospitals where babies are born must designate an expert in breastfeeding to carry out policies that benefit nursing mothers and babies. These include eliminating standing orders for antilactation drugs, letting infants nurse immediately after birth, not giving supplemental feedings unless they're specifically required for either the baby's or the mother's medical condition, letting babies nurse on demand, distributing discharge packs of infant formula only when specifically requested by mother or doctor, and educating new mothers on breastfeeding.

Hospitals *can* change and be more humane, in response to demands from patients and medical and nursing professionals. If you have a choice of hospitals in your community, ask about regulations and policies, and go with the one that offers more family-centered services. The more patients ask for these services, the more hospitals will offer them.

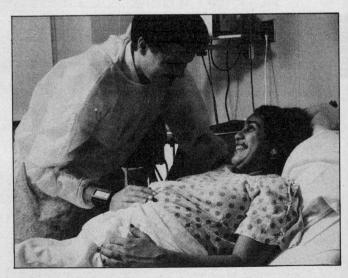

Sharing the birth experience with a supportive partner can help to get you through labor more comfortably.

The big plus of a hospital birth is that, should any complications occur, you will have an array of modern technology and professionals. If your pregnancy is considered high-risk, you'll certainly want to give birth in the hospital. If, as usually happens, your birth proceeds smoothly, you may be able to go home within 12 to 24 hours.

Even if your hospital does not have such policies, you can still have a good experience. Ask your doctor to leave written instructions that permit you to nurse your baby within one hour of birth; to have your baby brought to you on demand, including the middle of the night; not to give her any bottles of water or formula; and any other procedures that will help launch a successful course of breastfeeding. And even if your hospital stay does not go the way you'd like it to, remember that you'll be there for only a short time and that many women have overcome less than ideal hospital practices to go home and embark upon long and happy breastfeeding experiences.

•**Maternity Center/Birthing Center.** These free-standing centers offer a happy compromise between the comfort of home and the security of a well-equipped medical facility. They're usually staffed principally by nurse-midwives, with one or more physicians and nurse-assistants. They are designed for low-risk, uncomplicated births and offer prenatal care, birth in a homelike setting, and discharge the same day. Should complications arise, patients are transferred to a hospital. The most vital information to find out about a birth center are its staffing and its provision of emergency back-up services (contract with an ambulance service, agreement with a nearby reputable hospital, and on-premises emergency equipment).

•**Home Birth.** Over the past few years, some women who have access to a hospital have instead chosen to have their babies at home. They prefer to be in familiar surroundings, with family and friends and their older children, and to treat the birth as a normal family event. These births are often staffed by certified nurse-midwives or lay midwives, but there are also some physicians who strongly believe in the benefits of home births and assist in them.

If the pregnancy is low-risk and the birth uncomplicated,

this can work fine. It's often impossible to predict a sudden emergency during childbirth, however, and therefore it's vital to have back-up plans in case of emergency for quickly transporting mother and baby to a medical facility. This means that your home should be no more than 10 minutes away from the hospital and that previous arrangements should have been made with physician and hospital in case their services are needed. Obviously, it's especially important to check out the qualifications of your obstetric care provider if you're planning to have your baby at home.

PRENATAL CLASSES

No matter whom you choose as a practitioner and where you decide to bring your baby into the world, both you and your husband will benefit from enrolling in a prenatal education course. If you're a single parent or if your husband cannot or chooses not to attend, another supportive person (such as a mother, sister, or friend) can sign up with you to learn how to coach you during labor and delivery. Besides teaching techniques to help you during the birth, these classes help you plan your delivery, familiarize you with hospital procedures, and teach you how to get started with breastfeeding. Some hospitals also give courses to prepare children for the birth of a new sibling, to prepare grandparents for the birth of their grandchildren, and to educate couples expecting a second cesarean birth. To find out what's available in your community, you can call the obstetric department of a local hospital or contact ASPO/Lamaze or the International Childbirth Education Association (ICEA). See page 56.

PREPARING YOUR BREASTS

Most women around the world don't do anything at all to prepare their breasts for nursing; yet they breastfeed with hardly any problems. In our country, however, a number of routines are often recommended. Some of them do seem helpful, some actually hinder successful nursing, and some don't seem to make much difference one way or the other. Check with your

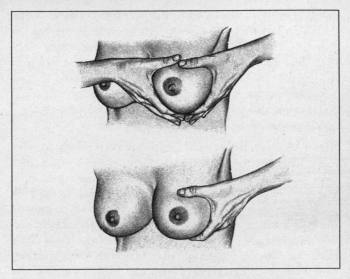

While it's not necessary to massage the breasts before delivery, some women find it helpful. To do it, twice a day circle one breast with the fingers and thumb of one hand, then the other. Close your hands together gently, about 10 times around the outer area and then about 10 times midway between the outer area and the areola. Repeat with the other breast.

obstetrician before doing any nipple stimulation during pregnancy.

Measures to avoid absolutely are rubbing the nipples with a nail brush to toughen them or applying alcohol, witch hazel, or tincture of benzoin to harden them. These drying agents irritate the nipples and predispose them to cracking and pain. In fact, during the last two or three months of pregnancy and while you're nursing, you should not even use soap on your nipples. The glands on and around the nipples will be secreting substances to keep them clean, so there's no need for soap, which can dry them out.

Toughening the Nipples During Pregnancy. The breasts of the average bra-wearing American woman are so well protected that her nipples are not used to any friction at all and may become quite tender when the baby starts to suck. While there's no proof that the practices suggested in the box on page 68 (Ways to Toughen the Nipples) prevent nipple problems, they probably can't hurt—and some women feel they help. If they do nothing else, they help you get used to handling your breasts so that you'll feel more comfortable when you're doing this with your baby. Before you do any prenatal nipple preparation, check with your own doctor.

Breast Massage. Breast massage has not been proven to be of real value, but some women and doctors swear by it and since there's no evidence that it's harmful, you may want to do it. Its purpose is to bring the colostrum from the alveoli to the milk pools under the areolae and to stretch and prevent clogging of the milk ducts. It may also improve circulation and help prevent engorgement of the breasts after birth. Twice a day, circle the breast with the fingers and thumbs of both hands and then close them together gently, first about 10 times around the outer area and then about 10 times midway between the outer area and the areola.

Manual Expression of Colostrum. Prenatal hand-expression of the colostrum is also said to open the milk ducts and prevent engorgement, although we're not convinced that it really makes any difference. Also, since no one yet knows whether there's a fixed amount of colostrum in the breasts or whether it replaces itself, there's a chance that this valuable substance may be wasted through hand-expression. The major benefit of prenatal expression seems to be the chance it gives you to learn how to express milk before your baby is born. Later on, you may want to express milk to relieve engorgement or to supply milk if your baby is premature or if you'll be away from your baby for an extended period of time. Expressing only a drop or two at a time before birth will enable you to learn the technique without wasting the colostrum. After your milk supply is established, you'll be able to express or pump several ounces of milk at a time. (See the Appendix for instructions on hand-expression).

Inverted Nipples. This is one condition for which prenatal preparation seems to be clearly of value. To determine whether one or both nipples are inverted, perform this little test. Hold your breast at the edge of the areola between your thumb and forefinger and press in firmly but gently, while at the same time pulling your fingers away from each other. (You can also do this with the thumbs from each hand.) If the nipple seems to disappear within the flesh of the breast, it is inverted.

Usually nipples like this protrude normally by the end of the pregnancy, and in almost all cases they come out fully when the baby starts to nurse. Occasionally, however, they remain inverted and pose a real problem to the baby who cannot

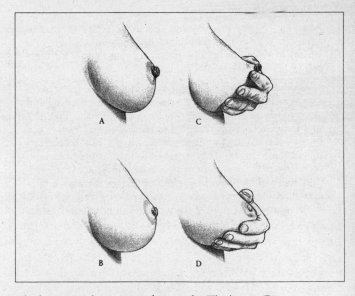

The breast (A) has a protruding nipple. The breast (B) is flat. To tell whether it is inverted, hold it at the edge of the areola between your thumb and forefinger. Press in firmly but gently, while at the same time pulling your fingers away from each other. This will either make it protrude as in (C) or invert as in (D).

Ways to Toughen the Nipples

• With a textured washcloth or towel, rub your nipples briskly but gently during or just after your daily shower or bath.

• For a few minutes every day (or longer, depending on your schedule and the level of privacy in your daily life), walk around the house with your breasts uncovered, to expose your nipples to the air.

• Allow your nipples to rub against your clothing occasionally, either by going without a bra, by cutting a little hole in your bra around the nipple area, or by wearing a nursing bra with the flaps down.

• As part of your lovemaking, encourage your husband to stimulate your breasts both manually and orally. There's no reason why you can't enjoy preparing your breasts for nursing.

• Some women find it helpful to do the simple exercise of nipple rolling once or twice a day. Do this after bathing and after you have rubbed the nipples with a towel. Take the nipple between your thumb and forefinger and pull it out firmly—just enough so that you feel it but not enough so that it really hurts. Then twist or roll the nipple between your fingers for a minute or two. Afterwards, apply a lubricant like pure lanolin (if you're not allergic to wool), vitamin A & D ointment, Massé cream, or salad or baby oil to the areola and the sides of the nipple—but not over the duct openings. Don't wipe off the cream or oil.

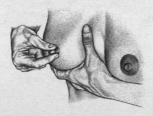

Nipple rolling

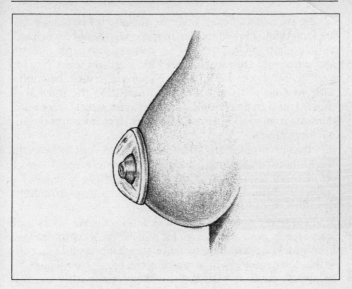

*Plastic breast shields (milk cups)[1] worn during
pregnancy often bring out inverted nipples.*

grasp the breast with her mouth. Fortunately, such a condition
is almost always correctable.

The "nipple-rolling" exercise described in the box on the
facing page sometimes helps. "Nipple pulling" (the Hoffman
technique) can also be useful. This involves grasping the nipple between your thumb and forefinger, drawing it forward,
and holding it there for a few seconds. Both of these can be
done twice a day at first; this exercise can eventually be performed more frequently.

By far the most successful treatment, however, is wearing
special plastic breast shields during pregnancy.[1] These shields,
also known as "milk cups," exert a constant, gentle, and painless pressure that gradually draws out a flat or inverted nipple.

[1]These shields/cups are made by several manufacturers. You may be able to
find them in your local drugstore or childbirth education organization. Some
of the trade names are Netsy, Woolwich, Confi-Dri, Mary Jane, Nurse-Dri,
Free and Dry, Hobbit, and Egnell/Ameda breast shells.

(These are quite different from the rubbery breast shields that are sometimes advised for sore nipples, but should *not* be used, as we explain in Chapter 7.) They come in two parts, fit easily into a bra, and are easy to wash with soap and water. Start to wear them about the middle of your pregnancy, beginning with an hour a day and gradually increasing the interval. If they fill up with colostrum, empty them frequently since warm moisture is an ideal setting for the growth of infection-causing microorganisms.

If your nipples are still inverted after birth, wear the shields between feedings, again being sure to empty them often. Do not feed the milk they trap to your baby unless you collect it within 15 minutes, as during pumping or expressing, described in the Appendix.

You won't need to wear these shields forever—only until your nipples protrude enough for nursing to occur. Since your baby's suckling will help to make this happen and since she will become more expert at grasping the breast, you'll probably be able to do away with the shields after the early stages of nursing. Once it is well established, you can start to "wean" yourself from the shields by going without them for a couple of hours before one of the midday nursings, not one for which your baby is apt to be frantically hungry. If the baby seems to have trouble nursing, go back to them for a while longer.

DEVELOPING YOUR SUPPORT NETWORK

In many countries around the world, mothering the new mother is taken for granted. There are plenty of people who are nearby to help her recover from childbirth and to care for her baby. In the United States today, the key word for most women is *independence*. You may live far away from the relatives and friends who would ordinarily help you. Or you may feel that you need to prove your adulthood, your womanhood, or your maternal competence by doing everything yourself. This puts a tremendous amount of pressure on you at a time when you need all the help you can get.

Anthropologist Dana Raphael has found that receiving help from a specific person or persons for a definite period of time after childbirth can go far in helping a mother with breastfeeding. She has coined the term *doula* for the person who gives such help. Before your baby is even born, you can look for the person(s) who will be *your* special helper(s).

Who will your special helper be? It could be one or more of these people in your life: your mother or mother-in-law, your father or sister, your husband or boyfriend, a friend or neighbor, your midwife, your doctor, a member of a breastfeeding support group like La Leche League, or your childbirth educator. Or it could be another new mother or a more experienced one whom you meet at your doctor's office, at the hospital, in a workshop for new or expectant parents (given in many communities by family service agencies or other social welfare organizations), or in a babysitting co-op. If you're planning to go back to work, try to find another working mother.

Given the fact that a formalized structure for giving such help doesn't normally exist in our society, you may have to seek out your own helpers. Raise your questions about breastfeeding and parenthood with the people who might be able to help you. Find out who you'll be able to count on for support, and how much each is able and willing to give. You'll also find out who to stay away from for a while.

When you identify the person or persons you feel most comfortable with, see if you can ask for the particular kinds of help you think you'll need most. This might involve asking him or her to come over for a couple of hours a day to help with household chores while you take care of the baby, to take care of the baby while you catch up on sleep, or to help you care for your baby by making suggestions on calming him when he's crying or holding her for nursing. Or it may involve nothing more than knowing you can phone your helper at any time of the day or the night with questions about child care or breastfeeding in particular. Depending on who the person is, you can work out some means of reciprocating this help, either now or in the future.[2]

---

[2]For helpful guidelines on finding and working out a relationship with a special helper, see *The Tender Gift: Breastfeeding,* by Dana Raphael (Schocken, 1973).

You'll need the most help in the first few weeks after your baby is born, the time period that's most crucial for the success of breastfeeding. If you can't find anyone to count on, you may have to be your own special helper, with the help of books to give you basic information and your telephone to contact resources. Whatever your situation, though, when questions come up, don't just stew over them privately. If you try hard enough, you'll be able to come up with answers.

LEARNING BREASTFEEDING TECHNIQUES

Breastfeeding is not an instinct; it is a learned skill. Most women get their first "hands-on" experience when they have their first baby. While most women and babies do, of course, master the techniques and quickly become a nursing couple, sometimes problems arise when a mother who doesn't know what to do holds a baby who doesn't know what to do either. You might feel more confident if you do a little practicing ahead of time.

You can do this with a soft doll about the size of a newborn baby. If you take a prenatal class, your instructor probably has such a doll. If you'd rather hold a real baby instead of a doll and if you have a friend currently nursing a baby, you may be able to visit her just before a feeding. She can let you hold her baby, who already knows what to do. This way you can get a feel for what it will be like when you will be holding your own baby. If you do this at a time when your friend's baby isn't extremely hungry, he'll probably be patient enough to spend a few moments in your arms before you turn him over to his mother for nursing.

One of the most exciting breastfeeding developments in recent years has been a new emphasis on positioning nursing babies. By videotaping breastfeeding mothers and their babies, researchers at the University of California were able to identify differences in the ways that mothers whose nursing was going well held their babies, compared to mothers who were either troubled by sore nipples or whose babies were not

Packing Your Bag

About six weeks before your due date you'll want to pack a small bag containing the items you want to take with you to the hospital or birth center. Among the items you may want to include:

•**A Nursing Bra.** Buy one in your eighth month of pregnancy. Your breasts are likely to be almost the same size they'll be while you're breastfeeding, so if you allow yourself a little room (as suggested in Chapter 5), it may fit after your milk comes in and will give you something to start out in. Some hospitals supply halter-type garments. While your own bras are more attractive, the hospital launders its supplies but not your personal items. So the choice of beauty or convenience is up to you.

•**A Nursing Nightgown.** This will have hidden side slits on the bodice. You'll look prettier than you would in those one-size-fits-all less-than-flattering hospital gowns and you'll have it to wear at home.

•**A Few Pairs of Underpants.** Whatever you wore while you were pregnant—bikini or maternity pants—will still fit since it takes a while to regain the waistline you once knew.

•**Telephone Numbers.** These should be for your childbirth educator, your obstetric care provider (so you can call your doctor in the office, for example, instead of trying to catch him or her in the hospital), and a local La Leche League leader so you can reach them easily if you have questions.

•**Your Favorite Books about Pregnancy and Breastfeeding.** Questions will arise and it's good to have something to refer to. You may even want to present a copy of a breastfeeding book to the nurses when you leave. They're apt to appreciate it more than a box of candy, since it will help them do their job better—and it isn't fattening.

gaining well. Thus, new technology has enabled us to learn new techniques for this age-old art.

Now your preparations are made and you're ready to embark upon one of the most challenging growth experiences of your entire life, parenthood. It's full of questions, worries, anxieties, satisfactions, thrills, and joy. Sound like a roller coaster? Hold on—and enjoy the ride!

5

The Care
and Feeding
of the
Nursing Mother

As a nursing mother you take it for granted that you need to take care of your baby. You may not realize, however, how much taking care of your baby depends on taking care of yourself, as well. Your health, your energy level, your comfort, and your state of mind all affect your ability to give milk. In addition, you need to remember that elements in your milk, such as drugs that you take recreationally or medicines that are prescribed for you, also reach your baby. (See Chapter 6.)

Above and beyond these considerations, you are not living *solely* for your baby even during these months. You have other people in your life, like your husband, your other children, other family members, and friends. Furthermore, you're still a person with your own life and your own needs. Ignoring those needs can have negative ramifications for you and for those you love, both now and in the years to come. For all these reasons, you want to pay attention to your own care while you're caring for your baby.

DIET:
WHAT YOU SHOULD
EAT AND DRINK

Just as you "ate for two" during pregnancy, you continue to "eat for two" during the time when most or all of your baby's food intake comes from your body. This does not, of course, mean that you eat twice as much as you normally eat. It does mean that, for your baby's optimal development, both before and after birth, your diet should contain essential nutrients throughout your entire pregnancy.

During pregnancy what you eat reaches your unborn baby in the form of the nutrients essential for growth and development. The first three months constitute the crucial period for the formation of the baby's organs; during the next three months, its body continues to grow and develop; and during the last three months of pregnancy, the baby is growing incredibly fast, with correspondingly high nutritional needs. The way a baby is nourished during these last months determines whether or not he'll be energy-deprived after birth. Take the vitamin supplements your doctor may prescribe, but do not make the mistaken assumption that they can replace a well-balanced diet. Supplements do not supply the necessary carbohydrates, protein, and fat that are found in food. Most of your vitamins and minerals should come from the grocery store, not the drugstore.

If you were eating well before you became pregnant, you won't have to make any changes during the first three months of your pregnancy; only moderate increases in your food intake will be necessary for the rest of the pregnancy and for the first three months of lactation. However, American teenagers and young women have notoriously poor eating habits. If your normal diet consists of a cigarette and coffee for breakfast, no lunch, and a fast-food dinner, this is a good time to mend your ways. Both you and your baby will benefit.

Over the past few years American eating habits have undergone a number of changes. Many of us have become more nutrition-conscious, and in line with our new awareness we have been eating more fresh vegetables and fruits, more fish, pasta, and grains, and less red meat, whole milk, and eggs. All

The Woman's Daily Food Guide

The following amounts represent *minimum* amounts of various foods that you should eat every day to get enough nutrition. You need more food than listed in this chart to get enough calories. For more detailed information on specific foods and serving sizes, see the box on page 78 (Food Guide During Pregnancy and Lactation).

FOOD GROUP	USUAL STATE	DURING PREGNANCY	WHILE NURSING
Protein Foods (lean meat, poultry, fish, eggs, or vegetable or grain equivalents)	2 servings	3 servings	3 servings
Dairy Foods (milk, yogurt, cheese)	2 cups (1 pint)	4 cups (1 quart)	4 cups (1 quart)
Breads and Cereals (including pasta, noodles, and rice)	4 servings	4 servings	4 servings
Fruits and Vegetables (1 serving each of vitamin A-rich and vitamin C-rich foods, and 2 other fruits or vegetables)	4 servings	4 servings	4 servings
Fats and Oils	2 tablespoons	2 tablespoons	2 tablespoons
Total Calories (for woman 5′4″, weighing 120 pounds)	1,700–1,900	2,000–2,200	2,200–2,400

This chart has been adapted from "Nutrition during Lactation," by Frances Stout, M.S., R.D., Nutrition Consultant, presented at the conference, "Strategies for Successful Breastfeeding," held at Beth Israel Medical Center in New York City on April 24, 1985.

Food Guide During Pregnancy and Lactation

FOOD GROUP		SERVINGS DAILY

PROTEIN FOODS	Pregnancy 3	Lactation 2

Choose From:

Lean cooked fish, meat, or poultry	2 ounces (after cooking)
Eggs	2
Dried beans or peas	1 cup cooked
Cheddar cheese	2 ounces
Cottage cheese	½ cup
Macaroni and cheese	1 cup
Chili with meat and beans	¾ cup
Cheese pizza	¼ of 14″ pie
Peanut butter	¼ cup
Nuts	½ cup
Seeds	½ cup
Tofu (soybean curd)	1 cup

CALCIUM SOURCES	Pregnancy 4	Lactation 4

Choose From:

Milk[1] (may be whole, skim, evaporated, dry, or buttermilk; may be used in soups, vegetables, or puddings)	1 cup
Yogurt	1 cup
Cheddar cheese	1½ ounces

[1]Milk is an excellent source of both calcium and protein. If you don't like or can't tolerate milk, you can obtain both these nutrients from other sources. However, if you don't drink the amount of milk recommended here, you need to increase your intake of protein above the amounts recommended.

Canned salmon or sardines (with bones)	3 ounces
Cottage cheese	2 cups[2]
Ice cream	1¾ cups[2]
Tofu	1 cup
Dried beans	3 cups cooked[2]
Kale, mustard, collard, or turnip greens	1 cup cooked
Broccoli	1 cup cooked

BREADS AND CEREALS (whole-grain preferable)	Pregnancy 4	Lactation 4

Choose From:

Bread	1 slice
Cornbread	1 square
Hamburger roll	½
Rice or grits	½ cup
Pasta or noodles	½ cup
Cooked cereal	½ cup
Ready-to-eat cereal	1 cup
Corn tortilla	1
Pizza crust	2½" wedge
Muffin	1 small
Wheat germ	1 tablespoon
Crackers	4

FRUITS AND VEGETABLES RICH IN VITAMIN A	Pregnancy 1	Lactation 1

Choose From:

Vegetables: broccoli, spinach, kale, greens, pumpkin, winter squash, sweet potatoes, carrots, asparagus, green pepper	1 cup raw or ¾ cooked

[2]These foods are not good sources of calcium; you would have to eat the large amounts shown here to get the same calcium as in 1 cup of milk).

(Continued on the next page)

Fruits: cantaloupe, peaches, watermelon	1 cup raw or ¾ cooked	

RICH IN VITAMIN C	Pregnancy 1	Lactation 1

Choose From:

Orange	1 medium
Grapefruit	½
Orange or grapefruit juice	4 ounces
Strawberries	½ cup
Cantaloupe	¼ melon
Broccoli	1 cup raw (¾ cup cooked)

GOOD IN VITAMIN C		

Choose From:

Green peppers	1 cup raw (¾ cup cooked)
Tomato	1 medium
Tomato juice	12 ounces
Tangerine	1 medium
Watermelon	½ cup
Coleslaw	½ cup

OTHER FRUITS AND VEGETABLES	Pregnancy 2	Lactation 2

FATS AND OILS	Pregnancy 2	Lactation 2

1 tablespoon		

The nutritional information in this chart has been adapted from "Nutrition during Lactation," by Frances Stout, M.S., R.D., Nutrition Consultant, presented at the conference, "Strategies for Successful Breastfeeding," held at Beth Israel Medical Center in New York City on April 24, 1985, and from E. R. Williams and M. A. Caliendo (1984). *Nutrition: Principles, Issues, and Applications.* (New York: McGraw-Hill).

these changes are in line with the guidelines for sound nutrition during pregnancy and lactation presented in the chart on page 78.

The foods listed in the box on the page 77 (The Woman's Daily Food Guide) don't cover all your calorie needs, so you'll need to add to them. You can calculate your own calorie needs by figuring out the amount that keeps you at a stable, normal weight, and then adding 300 calories for the latter half of pregnancy and 500 during lactation. For example, a woman 5'4" tall, who normally weighs 120 pounds, probably needs about 2,200–2,400 calories a day while she's breastfeeding.

Eat foods that have a high proportion of nutrients for the calories contained. "Empty calories"—foods that fill you up without fulfilling your nutritional needs—rob both you and your baby. You can eat the right kinds of foods and enjoy them, too, with flexible dietary guidelines. To be sure you're eating right for *you*, consult your doctor (or a registered dietitian or a nutritionist with a graduate degree in nutrition) and become knowledgeable about nutrition in general.

•No one food is indispensable. If you're allergic to eggs, substitute an ounce of meat or cheddar cheese, one-fourth cup of cottage cheese, or two tablespoons of peanut butter. If you hate milk or are lactose-intolerant, get equivalent nutrients by eating yogurt, cheese, and calcium-rich foods like broccoli and bone-in sardines.

•Calcium is a very important element in women's diets since it prevents *osteoporosis*, a thinning of the bones that causes widow's humps and fractures later in life. As a nursing mother, you need to be extra careful about getting enough calcium, since so much leaves your body in your milk. Be sure to get enough vitamin D (either through sunlight or a supplement), which helps you to absorb the calcium in your diet.

•The diets of many Americans are deficient in fruits and vegetables. You should eat a minimum of one citrus fruit every day (a rich source of vitamin C) and one serving of a vitamin A-rich fruit or vegetable (the darker the green vegetable or the deeper the orange of the squash, the more vitamin A). Increase your intake of leafy greens.

•Most American diets are too heavy in fat and added sugar, and too light on complex carbohydrates (breads, grains, and vegetables). You should be getting at least half of your calories from carbohydrates, about 30 to 35 percent from fat, and the rest from protein. To lose weight, you may find it easier if you decrease your fat intake to 25 to 30 percent of total calories.

•The food guide on page 78 provides a generous amount of protein (from the protein foods, milk, and bread), which you need during pregnancy and lactation. Notice that the serving portions for meat, poultry, and fish are much smaller than those served in most restaurants. The two-ounce servings recommended go far toward providing you with protein, while letting you save money and calories.

•Next to human milk, eggs contain the most usable protein in the human diet. More than half the protein is in the white, which has no fat or cholesterol (both of which are abundant in the yolk). While you can eat as many egg whites as you want, it's probably best not to eat more than four yolks a week, including those you use in cooking. In some recipes, for half the eggs called for, you can substitute two whites for one whole egg.

•To economize, substitute nonfat dry milk for liquid milk; take more of your protein in low-priced beans and grains than in meats; when you do buy meat get the cheaper cuts, which are often just as healthy; and buy fruits and vegetables in the cheapest form—fresh, frozen, or canned.

•To be sure you get enough iron, eat some of your protein in the form of lean red meats and organ meats (liver and heart). Meats are very rich sources of zinc and of iron in a readily absorbable form. You can improve your iron intake by eating iron-fortified cereals, cooking acidic foods like tomato sauce in cast-iron pots, and eating vitamin C-rich foods along with iron-rich foods to improve iron absorption (in combinations like orange juice and iron-fortified cereal or meatballs with tomato sauce). If you drink a lot of tea, you may want to take it between meals, since large quantities taken at mealtimes may interfere with the absorption of iron.

Your extra 500 calories a day, in addition to calories drawn from your body fat stores, should last you through the first six months of breastfeeding. If you nurse longer than that, your body fat stores may be diminished (especially if you have lost considerable weight), and your baby's growing nutritional needs may mean that you have to increase your caloric intake to make enough milk. If you're nursing twins or a very big baby, you may need to eat more.

By and large, you can be guided by your own body. If you're underweight to begin with or if you're very active, you may need more calories. If you're very overweight, you may have enough fat stores so that you can make do with fewer calories. After you start to nurse, you shouldn't be putting on weight—if you are, you're probably eating too much. If you're losing a great deal (more than one pound a week or two pounds a month), you should be eating more. You should not be losing weight rapidly, as we'll explain soon.

The Vegetarian Diet

If you're among the growing number of people who have eliminated meat from their diet, you know that a vegetarian diet can provide a healthful alternative if you choose your foods carefully and eat them in the best combinations. As a vegetarian nursing mother, you'll probably have a lower level of chemical pollutants in your breast milk, since many of these chemicals enter the body in animal fat.

However, since your needs for protein, vitamins, and minerals are higher when you're pregnant and nursing, you have to be especially aware of your food choices and the way to combine vegetable proteins to make them complete.[3] You also have to be sure to eat enough food, since plant products are lower in calories than animal foods. This is especially true for

---

[3]A comprehensive guide to doing this is *Diet for a Small Planet* by Frances Moore Lappe (1982). New York: Ballantine. Good information is also given in A. Eisenberg, H. Murkoff, and S. Hathaway (1986). *What to Eat When You're Expecting*. New York: Workman.

very strict vegetarians who eat no animal foods of any kind (*vegans*). Those who eat no meat, fish, or poultry, but do eat eggs and dairy products (*ovolactovegetarians*) or dairy products alone (*lactovegetarians*) have an easier time getting all their nutrients. People on these diets, however, sometimes eat large quantities of cheese as meat substitutes, not realizing that many cheeses contain more fat than most meats. You would do well to consult a registered dietitian or a nutritionist with a graduate degree in nutrition during these stages of your life to be sure that you're meeting your baby's nutritional needs, as well as your own.

While you're eating for two your daily needs will include six or more servings of grains, legumes, nuts, and seeds in combinations that provide complete proteins; three or more servings of vegetables (one or more dark leafy greens); one to four pieces of fruit (one citrus); and two or more glasses of milk or its calcium and protein equivalent. You may need supplements that include modest amounts of vitamin B_{12}, vitamin D, calcium, iron, zinc, and perhaps folic acid.

While adults can meet their bodies' needs even on a very strict vegetarian diet, infants and young children usually need some animal sources of protein to stay healthy and grow properly. Protein-calorie malnutrition, vitamin B_{12} deficiency, rickets (vitamin D deficiency), and growth retardation (due to insufficient zinc, protein, and calories) have been seen among some vegan children. For this reason, you may want to consider modifying your diet temporarily to eat eggs and dairy products throughout pregnancy and lactation, and you should add some animal protein sources to your children's diet after six months of age (even if you continue to breastfeed) until they're about five or six years old.

If you have been a vegan for several years, your breastfed baby should get vitamin B_{12}. Your baby may also need vitamin D if you live in a climate in which you or your baby cannot get enough exposure to sunshine. This is especially important if you're black, since recent research has found that some black women secrete less vitamin D in their milk than do white women.

Fluid Intake

Liquids are important in the diet, especially for the nursing mother, since you lose fluid in your milk. A cup of water, milk, soup, or fruit juice should become part of your routine before each nursing. While you may drink coffee, tea, and alcoholic beverages in moderation, don't depend on them to meet your body's needs for fluids, since they have a diuretic effect on some people. That is, they stimulate the kidneys to excrete more fluid, and so less liquid stays in the system.

Nursing women are sometimes urged to drink large quantities of liquids, but recent research on the effects of supplemental fluids doesn't show that they have any effect on increasing milk production. The most sensible approach, then, is to pay attention to your body's demands and to drink to satisfy your thirst.

You'll probably find that you become thirstier while you're nursing. If your urine seems very concentrated, you probably need to increase your fluid intake. You shouldn't be feeling overfull or bloated, though. If you are, you may be drinking too much. Too much fluid (more than 12 glasses a day) may slow your milk production. Since new mothers are often so busy that they disregard their bodies' signals, a good rule of thumb is to shoot for 6 to 8 glasses of fluid a day (including milk, juice, and other beverages).

LOSING WEIGHT: HOW MUCH, HOW SOON?

There's a paradox about nursing and women's weight. Breast-feeding does not make women gain weight. In fact, it uses up calories and therefore helps to get rid of extra weight. Nature's way of providing the extra calories needed for milk production is to store up fat during pregnancy. Then lactation helps to use up these fat stores. Therefore, the nursing mother is more likely to lose the weight she gained during her pregnancy than is the woman who does not nurse her baby. However, this loss of weight is apt to come later for the nursing mother than it is for the non-nursing woman, who can begin to diet safely sooner after childbirth.

If you're breastfeeding, there are several reasons why you should not be dieting strenuously. First, your body needs to have enough nutrients to produce the milk. If you cut down too drastically on what you eat, you'll be robbing your body. It will maintain the quality of the milk at your expense by cutting into your lean tissues (your muscles), your bones, and your blood cells. This means that you could lose muscle tone, bone density, and blood strength. Then, if you become very undernourished, you'll produce less milk. Another major argument against crash dieting during lactation is the concentration of environmental pollutants in fat cells. When you lose a great deal of weight, the fat in the cells of your body breaks down quickly, releasing contaminants that have been stored in body fat into your milk.

Thus, you'll serve yourself and your baby best by *gradually* dropping any excess weight left over from your pregnancy. You can, of course, cut down without cutting out in a number of ways. You can substitute skim milk for whole milk; broil, boil, roast, or bake meats and potatoes instead of frying them; eat more fish and poultry; avoid fatty meats and fish like pork and mackerel; snack on raw vegetables and fruits instead of potato chips and cookies; eat fresh fruits rather than sweetened canned ones; go lightly on high-calorie vegetables and fruits like avocados, cherries, and sweet potatoes; and stay far, far away from high-fat cheeses, rich sauces, fatty salad dressings, sugared soft drinks, sugary cereals, cookies, cakes, pastries, and candy.

A safe rule of thumb is to plan to lose no more than two and a half pounds per month while you're nursing. Thus, in six months you'll have lost 15 pounds and by eight months you'll have lost 20. This, in addition to the weight you lost with your baby's birth, will probably bring you back down to or close to your prepregnancy weight. Many women adopt the attitude that it took nine months to put on all those pounds, so it's not unrealistic to expect it to take the same amount of time to take them off.

This may happen without any special effort on your part, so you may want to wait for two or three months after childbirth and see what happens. Monitor your weight and if you're losing steadily, as some women do, you don't have to do anything special about your eating habits. If not, you can start to cut back gradually. Then by the time your baby is nine months old and is taking less milk in proportion to other foods in her diet, you can begin to plan to lose one to two pounds per week. Losing weight slowly by changing your eating habits and your exercise patterns is better than dropping it quickly, since you're more likely to keep the pounds off. A well-planned exercise schedule is extremely important in your weight-loss program for a number of reasons, which we'll talk about in more detail.

This stricture against losing considerable weight during lactation does not necessarily hold for women who are very overweight. One new mother we know had put on 30 excess pounds before she got pregnant and then gained another 50 pounds during her pregnancy. With the help of her doctor, she worked out a low-calorie balanced diet and over a period of eight months lost 65 pounds, with no apparent ill effects to her baby or herself. Because the effects of toxins may not show up for many years, such a large weight loss should be undertaken only if medically indicated for a woman's health.

Some women do, of course, lose the weight they gained during pregnancy very soon after their babies are born and remain quite slender throughout lactation and afterward. You don't have to be plump to be a good milk producer. Most women, however, need to think about their weight in a new way. When did you ever see a thin fertility symbol? Just as breastfed babies grow differently from formula-fed babies, the bodies of breastfeeding mothers follow a different schedule from those of non-nursing mothers. A substantial weight gain during pregnancy helps to assure a healthy baby, and part of that weight seems to be nature's way of providing milk after the baby is born.

If you're a typical contemporary American woman, you'll probably have no more than two or three children in your lifetime. Recognizing that your nutritional status has to support your life and your baby's and recognizing the very small proportion of time in relation to your total life span that breastfeeding takes, you need to ask yourself whether you can stand being a few pounds heavier after the birth of each baby, with the assurance that after you've stopped nursing it will be possible to lose this extra weight. Since you also recognize the value of breastfeeding to both of you, you can probably answer this question in the affirmative.

FOODS TO AVOID WHILE NURSING

If you have no food allergies yourself, most of the foods you eat won't cause problems for your baby. Some foods eaten by the mother do, however, seem to affect her baby adversely. A major offender for some women seems to be cow's milk. In a number of cases, nursing babies who had symptoms of colic (sharp intestinal pains, usually accompanied by gas) showed great improvement when their mothers stopped drinking cow's milk or eating cow's milk products. The same kind of result has shown up in babies with other symptoms, including vomiting, diarrhea, runny noses, wheezy bronchitis, and eczema. (If your baby is colicky and you stop drinking cow's milk for a while, try it again a couple of weeks later. It's possible that your baby's digestive system may have matured enough to handle the milk, and you won't need to deprive both of you of the good nutrients milk contains.)

Other foods that are implicated to a lesser extent include eggs, citrus fruits, wheat, and chocolate. Some allergists have commented that the foods babies react to are often those that the mothers had eaten in large amounts while she was pregnant, giving rise to the possibility that the baby may have been sensitized to them in utero.

Nursing babies sometimes suffer from gas after mothers eat foods from the cabbage family, such as broccoli or brussels sprouts. Others become crampy after their mothers drink herbal teas or wakeful after their mothers drink coffee or other foods containing caffeine such as tea, cola drinks, or chocolate. One nursing mother found that her baby got sick whenever she had eaten something with garlic in it, and then she remembered that her husband suffered cramps after eating garlic, making her think that they both might have the same kind of allergic reaction.

One case reported in the medical literature was that of a three-month-old baby whose urine was periodically a bright pink. After the mother noticed that she had trouble removing an orange-pink stain from a plastic glass from which she drank orange soda, she tried abstaining from this drink—and then trying it and watching the baby's urine. There seemed to be a definite connection, and so the mother eliminated the soda from her diet.

To minimize the risk of passing on environmental pollutants in your milk, you should avoid freshwater fish from waters known to be contaminated; peel or thoroughly wash fruits and vegetables to get rid of pesticide residues; cut away the fatty portions of meats, poultry, and fish (dark sections and skin), since chemicals tend to be concentrated in the fat; and avoid dairy products rich in butterfat.

Some foods eaten in large amounts give the milk a distinctive taste, which an occasional baby with a discriminating palate may not like, causing him to reject the breast milk. (It's estimated to take four to six hours between the time you eat the food and the time it affects your milk.) If you can establish any relationship between certain foods that you eat and reactions from your baby, it's easy enough to avoid these foods. For the most part, however, you can eat any nourishing food that you want without fear that your baby will be affected.

WHAT FOODS MAKE MILK?

Virtually every culture in the world has proffered certain foods to nursing mothers, in the belief that they help to make milk. In China, nursing mothers have been urged to eat "a mixture of pork fat and red gram, cuttlefish soup, shrimps' heads in wine, and a special sweet wine made from glutinous rice, given together with the larvae of the blow-fly." In India, garlic, tamarind, and cottonseed are customarily offered breastfeeding women. All over the world, herbal preparations are freely given to increase a mother's milk supply. Dr. Derrick B. Jelliffe, director of Population and Family Health at UCLA, has concluded that the effects of such potions are largely psychological. The mother thinks that a certain food will increase her milk supply, so she relaxes and has a good let-down reflex, "proving" the value of the food.

The best way to build up your milk supply isn't what *you* eat, though; it's what your baby eats. The more often you nurse your baby and the more vigorously she nurses, the more milk you're likely to have. (For other suggestions on building up your milk supply, see Chapter 7.)

EXERCISE:
HOW MUCH, HOW SOON?

The United States is in the midst of an exercise boom. The trendiest clothes around these days are running shoes, warm-up suits, and leotards, and as we go to press the Jane Fonda exercise videocassette has topped the best-seller lists for over three years and is the highest grossing videocassette ever published. This is particularly good news for nursing mothers, for both short-term and long-range reasons.

First of all, following a specific postnatal exercise program will help tone up sagging postpregnancy muscles, so that you'll feel and look better. It will help you avoid the backache that plagues so many new mothers, as you find yourself bending and lifting more than you've done in your entire life. And it will speed up your sexual recovery by tightening muscles that were stretched during childbirth.

Furthermore, exercise isn't only for the postpartum period. There's considerable evidence that exercise actually

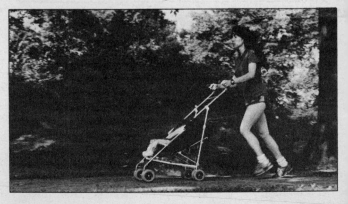

Jogging while pushing a stroller gives this mother her exercise and the baby her fresh air.

tends to diminish appetite while using up calories, so it's a vital element in maintaining desirable body weight. It helps you build your muscles, strengthen your heart and lungs, lower your blood pressure, protect against heart attacks and cancer, and possibly lengthen your life. Weight-bearing exercise like walking, running, jogging, and bicycling is effective in fat control, and it also helps to increase bone density, thus being an important aid to the prevention of osteoporosis. It's a better stress and anxiety reducer than tranquilizers and can, therefore, contribute to your mental health. And when you find an activity you like, it can actually be fun—even if you've always been one of those people who react to the urge to exercise by immediately lying down. The fun can be shared, too, as bicycling, skating, folk dancing, and various other vigorous activities form a good basis for lively family and other social outings.

Postpartum Exercise

You can begin to do some exercises within 24 hours after your baby is born if you start easy, build up gradually, and use common sense. For a specific program, see one of the books on pregnancy recommended in Chapter 4, and check your bookstore for books on exercise before and after childbirth.[4] You can start right away with pelvic tilts, Kegel exercises, and deep breathing. In a few days, you can move on to head and leg lifts, leg slides, and a variety of stretching and bending exercises.

Do not overdo it! You should warm up slowly, rest between exercises, and stop before you feel tired. Fatigue is an enemy of successful breastfeeding. At the beginning it's more important to establish your milk supply than to preserve your reputation as an athlete. If you develop any unusual symptoms, such as pain, increased vaginal bleeding, dizziness, faintness, or shortness of breath, stop and call your doctor.

---

[4]You can also get videotapes, audiotapes, and records that guide you through a 50-minute workout of calisthenics to music, specially designed for pregnant and newly delivered women. The program has been developed in cooperation with the American College of Obstetricians and Gynecologists. You can buy them in some doctors' offices, book and video stores, and maternity shops, or order them from Feeling Fine Programs, 3575 Cahuenga Blvd. West, Los Angeles, CA 90068, (800) 443-4040, ext. 161.

Exercise Guide
for the Nursing Mother

•Choose an activity that you enjoy doing, so that you'll keep on doing it. While you're nursing, you may want to avoid weight lifting or other strenuous exercises involving repetitive arm movements, since some women attribute clogged milk ducts to such activities. This still leaves a wide range of activities to choose from, including walking, running, jogging, cycling, folk-dancing, yoga, and jumping rope. (Swimming is notable here by its absence; while it's an excellent exercise for building muscles and body tone, it's not as effective as weight-bearing exercises for controlling fat and building bone density.)

•Try to find an "exercise buddy," a friend you can work out with two or three times a week. You'll stimulate each other to keep up with the program, and you'll make your workout do double duty as a social get-together. Don't fall into the trap of judging yourself by what your buddy can do, however.

•Concentrate on activities that you can do without leaving your baby or at times when someone else can be with the baby. This may mean exercising on a stationary bicycle or other at-home equipment, jumping rope, or working out with a videocassette. It may mean walking while carrying your baby in a backpack (an excellent way to use up more

The amount of exercise you do will vary, depending on how active you were before you gave birth. If you were very sedentary or if you're now anemic or very overweight, you should do only limited exercise, with your doctor's approval.

One way to monitor your progress is to keep a chart of the number and kinds of exercises you do each day. You'll be able to see how much more you can do as the days go by, and you'll feel proud of your efforts.

calories in your exercise program). Or it may mean running early in the morning or at night when your husband or older children are home.

•Schedule your exercise around your breastfeeding. Working out immediately after nursing the baby works best, since your breasts are not full and uncomfortable and the baby won't be hungry for a while. Some women nurse the baby first thing in the morning (sometimes even before the baby is fully awake), put her back to bed, and then do their exercise. One working mother told us about her late-night schedule: Three evenings a week, after nursing the baby at about 10:00 P.M., she runs for half an hour with a friend. This is the advantage of choosing an activity for which you don't have to meet anyone's schedule but your own.

•If your favorite exercise program involves going out to a class, treat yourself to a babysitter or trade off with a friend, so you can get to your class. It will do double duty as a social outing as well as a physical one.

•Dress comfortably. Wear a bra. If you're full-figured, a nursing bra may not provide enough support, so it pays to buy a sport bra in the larger size you need now and to change into it for your exercise sessions. Wear underpants that don't ride up, rub, or constrict. Cotton or polypropylene absorb sweat best. If you get overheated when wearing leotards and tights, switch to shorts and a T-shirt.

Developing a Regular Exercise Schedule

One 39-year-old woman we know, who has been running regularly for 14 years, ran eight miles a day before she became pregnant and continued to run during her pregnancy, cutting down her distance to two miles a day in late pregnancy. She has even done one last short run as her labor was beginning. Within one to two weeks after the birth of each of her five children she began running again. She has breastfed them all and has always produced plenty of milk. Why does she do it? Here's what she says: "I feel better overall if I exercise regularly. I run to stay fit and have a chance to be outdoors every day. Running helps control my appetite and weight and lets me eat more! It also sets a good example for the kids; by spells they run and participate regularly in various activities."

While just reading about this active a schedule will exhaust most of us, it's heartening to see that it can be done. And it clearly shows that less ambitious exercise programs are eminently feasible. The important thing is for you to figure out what you like to do and what's comfortable for you to do—and then to keep doing it on a regular basis. It's better to exercise three or four days a week, for about half an hour to an hour at a stretch, than to work out every day or on a sporadic, catch-as-catch-can basis.

The most important thing for you to realize is that you're doing the best thing you can for your baby by breastfeeding, and that, as one mother said, "I know that everything else I do is gravy." Eventually you'll lose your extra weight, you'll go back to your former measurements, and you'll be able to do more physically. For the duration of nursing, do what you feel good about doing and feel good about yourself. For suggestions for exercising while breastfeeding, see the box on page 92 (Exercise Guide for the Nursing Mother).

CARE OF YOUR BREASTS

While you're nursing you don't need to bother with any special nipple-care rituals. Be especially careful not to use any drying agents on them, including soap. If you splash water over the nipples during your daily shower and change your bra at least once a day (or more often, if you're leaking a great deal of milk), your nipples will be clean.

If the hospital nurse asks you to wash your nipples with sterile water before each feeding, go ahead and do it. It's not necessary, but it doesn't have any ill effects. If you're told to wash with a drying agent, however, don't do it just to be a "good" patient. This is one of those times when you need to be assertive. You can always say your doctor told you not to.

While breastfeeding women have for years been advised to apply a soothing ointment to the nipples after feedings to prevent or treat nipple soreness, research does not show any evidence that any of these creams or salves help. If it feels good to apply such over-the-counter preparations as plain lanolin, A & D ointment, or Massé cream, do it—they won't hurt you. Be sure to wipe them off gently before you nurse.

A more effective practice is keeping the nipples dry—changing bra or breast pad if they get wet from leaking milk and walking around with your nipples uncovered when you can to let air circulate around the nipples.

Most women experience some soreness, usually on the second or third day of nursing, but occasionally later. If you develop soreness that's more than mildly uncomfortable and if it doesn't go away in a day or two, treat it immediately as suggested in Chapter 12.

Wearing the Right Bra

This is probably the single most important item in your wardrobe these days. The nursing bra you bought at the end of your pregnancy may still fit after your milk comes in if you allowed a little extra room. If it's too tight, though, *do not wear it*, since a tight bra can cause clogged milk ducts and a great deal of discomfort. If you find you like this style after wearing it for a couple of weeks, you can order more by phone or ask someone else to pick them up for you. If not, look for a style you like better.

Even if you're small-breasted and don't ordinarily wear a

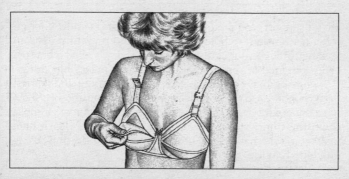

A comfortable nursing bra that lets you uncover one breast at a time, using only one hand, makes life—and nursing—easier.

A Few Beauty Tips for the Nursing Mother

•Make life as easy for yourself as possible. Find a few simple routines you can stick to and make them yours. It may be all you can do to run a comb through your hair and wash your face once a day.

•Custom-tailor your routine to your own priorities. Since you can't do everything you did before, pick the parts of you whose looks you care the most about—and take care of them. One woman, for example, may feel messy if she doesn't wash her hair every day; another can't stand seeing unpolished nails; a third feels unkempt with unshaven legs.

YOUR HAIR

•Don't make a radical change in the way you wear your hair, unless you're going from a very elaborate coif to a "wash-and-wear" one. Don't have a style that you need to set. Wait to get a permanent, since it may not take during or soon after pregnancy.

•If you hate the way your hair looks, put on a sweatband

bra for support, you'll probably want to wear one now if for no other reason than to hold breast pads or to prevent milk from leaking through your clothes. While you don't need a bra specially designed for breastfeeding, it usually makes life easier.

Nursing bras come in a wide variety of styles and fabrics, from no-nonsense sturdy to lacy and sexy. Some are soft; some have underwires for added support. Some have a row of hooks down the front; others have a hook at the top of each cup; look for a style that lets you uncover one breast at a time, using only one hand.

A properly fitted bra is important in maintaining your breast contours, so keep the following points in mind when you go shopping. The cup of the bra should support the entire lower half of the breast in a natural position. (With the bra on, that matches your sweatsuit, or a cap with a visor that matches your shorts.

YOUR SKIN

•Your skin may become coarser and blotchy during and soon after pregnancy. Be patient. This, too, will change.

•When you think of it, put some hand or body lotion or baby oil on your body. A loving way to ease back into intimacy with your husband is to give each other body massages. You can do this even if you don't feel ready to become sexually active.

YOUR NAILS

•You'll probably be more comfortable if your nails are short and pale rather than long and dark. Aside from the danger of scratching your baby, long nails are more likely to break. When bright red nail polish chips, it's more obvious than when a light one does. You may want to buff your nails now instead of polishing them.

•The fun place to apply polish these days is on your toenails. For one thing, it's wonderful to know that you can reach them again. For another, they won't chip so fast, and you might enjoy the undercover glamour.

hold your arms straight down at your sides. If it fits properly, the nipple line will be level with a point midway between elbow and shoulder.) The band should fit snugly, neither binding nor slipping up and down. To test this, put your hands on your hips and look at yourself, front and back, in the mirror. The straps should be broad and adjustable, and preferably padded or cushioned. The bra should not be so tight that it leaves marks in your skin under the arms, under the breasts, or over your shoulders.

When buying bras before your baby is born, allow for a little growth after your milk comes in. You'll want a little bit of extra room in the cups and in the band, so be sure not to buy a size that you already have to wear on the loosest hook.

If you don't need the support of a more structured bra, you

may prefer to wear a simple stretch bra that can be easily pulled up for nursing rather than one designed specifically for breastfeeding.

You need at least three bras—one on you, one in the drawer, and one hanging up to dry. If you're leaking a great deal of milk, you'll want to change bras or liners often to keep your nipples from getting sore and your clothes from getting stained.

To absorb leaking milk, you can put some type of lining inside the bra. You can buy disposable nursing pads in the drugstore, but if you want to save money or if you find that they stick to your breasts, you can easily make your own pads. Insert a folded man's all-cotton handkerchief in each cup of your bra, or cut out four-inch circles from all-cotton diapers or old T-shirts and stitch three or four thicknesses together. (Synthetic fabrics and no-iron finishes are not as absorbent.) Be sure to change these breast pads often enough to keep your breasts dry. Milk-soaked pads that remain next to your skin form an ideal place for bacteria to grow, possibly causing sore nipples or a breast infection. Some women find that plastic milk cups, the kind used to bring out inverted nipples as described on page 69, are better for catching leaking milk. These need to be kept dry, too, and emptied often if you're leaking a great deal.

Leaking is usually common in the early weeks, but it stops being a problem within a couple of months. If you're still leaking through your clothes despite your precautions, try stopping it by pressing your breast with the heel of your hand or your forearm when you feel the tingling that signals let-down.

Lumps in the Breast

If you discover a lump in your breast while nursing or in your monthly self-examination, chances are that it is related in some way to the fact that you're breastfeeding. If it hurts, it may signal a plugged duct or an infection, which you'll treat by the methods suggested in Chapter 12. If it doesn't hurt, it may be a tumor. The likelihood is that such a tumor is benign, but it can be dangerous to ignore such a symptom. In any case, if you develop any lump that remains for more than three days, call your doctor.

You do not need to wean your baby before your breast examination, and even if you have to have the lump removed surgically, you may be able to continue nursing on the other side and eventually to resume nursing on the affected side.

GETTING ENOUGH REST

Weariness seems to be the lot of every new mother. Right after your body has undergone the aptly named experience of labor, you have more responsibilities but get less sleep. If stress and fatigue kept women from breastfeeding, none of us would be here today, because our mothers, grandmothers, and great-grandmothers and more distant forebears certainly had their

---

Ways to Guard Your Rest

THE TELEPHONE

Telephones are wonderful lines of communication, but they can also be invaders of privacy and disturbers of rest. They don't have to be, though, if you take precautions like the following:

•When you and the baby want to rest, turn off the bell on the telephone.

•Hook up an answering machine with a message along the lines of the following: "I'm sleeping or busy with the baby right now. Please leave your name and number and I'll call you back when I can." Or indicate when someone else will be home to answer the phone.

•Return the phone calls while lying in bed at a time when it's convenient for you to handle them.

THE DOORBELL

To prevent being disturbed by unexpected callers or solicitors, hang a notepad and pen on the door, next to a sign that says something like this: "Please do not ring the doorbell. Baby is sleeping. Please leave a note."

Clothes for the Nursing Mother

You probably don't need to buy anything special to wear while you're nursing. Most women already have enough suitable clothing to wear as is, or with minor alterations. However, if you do want to pick up a few extra wardrobe items, they may give your spirits a lift as you look good and enjoy extra convenience. Of course, you'll pick things that are washable and wrinkle-resistant and that don't need ironing.

•Warm-up suits or sweatsuits are ideal for your first postpartum wardrobe: They come in a range of wonderful colors and fabrics from terry to velour, the waistlines are adjustable, the pullover tops hide your thick middle when you're not nursing and can be easily pulled up when you are, you can keep them on while you sneak in a nap, and they're easy to throw into the washer and dryer. With coordinated socks, sneakers, barrettes, and/or headband, you can have a put-together look—and you'll look like an athlete even if you don't feel like one. If you can afford it, buying three or four in different colors will give you a basic everyday wardrobe, which you'll probably still be wearing after you've weaned your baby. (If you had a cesarean birth, with a midline incision, these would not be a good choice since you won't want anything elastic around your waist until the incision heals, so you probably don't want to go overboard on buying these until after your baby is born.)

•Nursing nightgowns, which also come in a range of styles and fabrics, are also good for both comfort and morale, although two-piece pajamas work well, too.

•For more formal occasions, separates—blouses, T-shirts, and other tops, worn with skirts or pants—are easier to manipulate than dresses. Wraparound skirts or skirts and pants with elasticized waists are especially good, since your former waistline will be only a fond memory for a few months.

•Button-front blouses are convenient, but so are knit pullovers, which can be easily pulled up to allow for modest nursing. When you're wearing a button-front blouse, you can nurse more discreetly if you unbutton from the bottom up rather than from the top down. When you wear a pullover, the baby's body will cover your midriff and the pullover will cover your breasts.

•Choose prints and colors that won't show milk that may leak through. Avoid white, pale colors and clingy materials.

•Ponchos and loose-fitting cardigan sweaters and jackets are good cover-ups for unobtrusive nursing.

•Breast pads that fit into your bra will absorb leaking milk and prevent your clothes from getting stained. You can make your own out of 3-inch squares cut from a plain white all-cotton T-shirt. They're very absorbent, fold to the size you need, wash and dry quickly, and don't show through. If you use disposable breast pads, try to get the kind with no gauze lining, since this can stick to your breasts and cause hairline cracks and painful tenderness. If you buy fabric pads, look for all-cotton ones, since synthetic fibers are not absorbent.

•You may want to have one pretty scarf or shawl that you can keep handy to drape around your shoulders when an unexpected caller comes to the door in the middle of a feeding.

•Don't try to squeeze into too-tight prepregnancy clothes. You'll look fat and poorly groomed, and you'll be uncomfortable (and probably depressed). Tight blouses rub against your nipples and can trigger a let-down at the most inconvenient times.

•A number of companies specialize in making clothes for nursing women. You can find their ads in the pages of magazines aimed at new mothers, and you can usually send away for catalogs and order the clothes by mail.

•If you sew, you can make your own clothes or adapt those you already own. You can, for example, make horizontal seams clear across the bustline or open up darts under it where you can insert invisible zippers. Or you can put zip-

(Continued on the next page)

pers under the armholes of sleeveless dresses. You can attach fake pockets over each breast with Velcro. A flip of your wrist will lift a corner of the pocket to make the breast accessible to the baby but protected from public view.

•If you work outside the home, see the suggestions in Chapter 9 for clothes for the working nursing mother.

---

share of both. However, the better you feel, the easier the breastfeeding will go, so it makes sense to get as much rest as possible.

If you can hire someone to help you in the house right after you come home from the hospital, the money you spend will be a wonderful investment that will yield dividends for the entire family. Maybe you can find a high school or college student or a mature person who can come in for a few hours each afternoon, straighten up the house, take your older children out, and cook and clean up after dinner. One new mother told us what a help it is to have someone come in for just one hour every other day, to put away laundry, to hang up clothes, to take out garbage, and to wash dishes.

If your budget doesn't allow this, perhaps the person or persons acting as your "doula," or special helper, can help out in some ways, for which you can reciprocate at some time in the future. Marketing, bringing a cooked meal, and taking out your older children are all tasks that friends and family members will often do cheerfully.

HOW YOU LOOK

Since how you look affects the way you feel, it's worthwhile to invest a little time, effort, and money into looking good. You're at a stage in your life that has inspired artists in every culture in every era in history.

The thought and care that you put into both the inner and the outer you will pay off in the success of your breastfeeding. The better you feel, the happier the experience is likely to be. And the better cared for you are, the more your baby will benefit.

6

Drugs and the Nursing Mother

From time immemorial people have taken a variety of drugs for a variety of reasons—to drown their sorrows, to ease their pain, to achieve new levels of consciousness. During the past several decades, however, our pharmacopoeia has mushroomed incredibly: 90 percent of all the medications available today were unknown 40 years ago. In addition, with advances in medical research we have learned that drugs taken by the mother can affect the fetus she's carrying in her womb and the baby she's breastfeeding.

While you're nursing your baby, you're justifiably concerned about anything that you take into your body. Your major questions are whether the particular agent will pass through your milk, and if it does, whether it will affect the baby. There's been a great deal of interest in this in recent years, as more women have been breastfeeding and more drugs have come on the market.

It's comforting to know that in general, most commonly used drugs can be taken safely by the nursing mother. In this chapter we'll pay the most attention to the effects of drugs on the nursing baby. If you are now pregnant it's absolutely essential for you to consult your doctor before you take any chemical agent. Some drugs, both over-the-counter and those prescribed by doctors, can have adverse effects on the fetus.

The basic rule of thumb, whether you're pregnant or nursing, is not to take any drug unless there is a sound medical reason for it. This is the best course for both you and your baby. If there is some medical indication, however, that a particular agent is important for your physical and emotional well-being, in *most* cases you can take it. See the boxes on the following pages (Drugs That Can Safely Be Taken by Nursing Mothers; Drugs That Require a Temporary Cessation of Breastfeeding; and Drugs That Should Not Be Taken by Nursing Mothers).

MEDICINES

There is a world of difference between pregnancy and lactation, as far as the ability of drugs to affect the infant. A number of medicines taken by the pregnant woman can cause serious birth defects in the developing fetus. On the other hand, most medicines taken by a nursing mother do not seem to harm her baby. Still, it's possible that some drugs that may be safe for a fetus, because the mother's kidney and liver act to detoxify chemicals, are not safe for a newborn baby whose own system is too immature to do this important task. We cannot, therefore, apply what we know about one state to the other.

In their 1984 report, Dr. Gregory White and Mary White have written: "Verified reports of a medication having actually harmed a nursing infant are still virtually nonexistent . . . the baby is nearly always unaffected by the medications taken by his mother." Those qualifiers "virtually" and "nearly," however, flash warning signals that in some cases such medications may pose risks.

The problem is that there's so much we don't know. We don't, for example, know about the long-term effects of a baby's receiving drugs through the mother's milk; we don't know whether receiving drugs now in infancy might cause a hypersensitivity to certain components later on; we don't know whether a buildup of the drug in the baby's system could cause problems; we don't know what kinds of conditions might show up in 10 or 20 or even more years.

What, then, are you to do right now? As an overriding rule of thumb (even for people who are not nursing an infant), it's best to take the least amount of medication that will be effective. If you don't *need* it, don't take it. If you do need it, there are ways to minimize its effects on your baby.

Whenever possible, it's better to continue breastfeeding than to wean a baby prematurely. This is especially true if the weaning would be abrupt. Sudden weaning is painful for the mother and upsetting for both mother and baby. Early weaning also deprives the baby of the benefits of breastfeeding. Therefore, it makes sense for mother and doctor to work together to solve medical problems within the context of breastfeeding.

Drugs That Can Safely Be Taken by Nursing Mothers

Medicines that breastfeeding mothers can generally take with safety in the usual doses and continue to nurse their babies are:

Acetaminophen
Antidepressants
Most antihistamines
Aspirin
Decongestants
Quinine
Tolbutamide (for diabetes)
Most vaccines
Most antibiotics

Antiepileptics
Antihypertensives
Codeine
Phenobarbital (in small amounts; doses large enough to put the mother to sleep make the baby sleepy, too)
Drugs that enhance thyroid function
Most tranquilizers

Sources for this and the boxes on pages 109 and 112: American Academy of Pediatrics Committee on Drugs, 1983; Sia, 1985; Govoni and Hayes, 1985. Names in parentheses after generic names of drugs are common trade names.

While the boxes on the following pages give recommendations for some common drugs, new ones are coming on the market every day and new findings are emerging about many established ones, so these lists are only guides at best. To assure your baby's health, follow these guidelines:

•You can take an occasional aspirin, antihistamine, or other mild over-the-counter preparation without checking first with your doctor. You should not be taking large amounts of these, nor should you take anything over a long period of time without your doctor's knowledge. (This is important for your own health, too; you may be masking symptoms of a serious nature.)

•Before taking any new drug, check with *your baby's* doctor, as well as with the one prescribing the drug for you. Tell your doctor or dentist—whoever is prescribing the medicine—that you are nursing your baby. Ask the following questions:

1. What complications or discomfort would result from *not* taking the drug? Would they be acceptable, from both medical and comfort standpoints? Would it be safe for you to forego treatment? You could probably put up with a few aches and pains, but if your health is at stake, being a martyr will benefit neither you nor your baby.

2. Can you safely postpone treatment until your child is older and his system is better able to detoxify chemicals in the milk? Sometimes a compound that would be dangerous for a one-week-old or one-month-old poses no problem for an older baby.

3. Does this drug pass through the breast milk? Most drugs do, so that the baby gets about 1 to 2 percent of the mother's dosage, but usually this is not dangerous.

4. Is this drug potentially dangerous to your baby? (Ask your doctor the question posed by Ruth Lawrence, M.D., in her book, *Breast Feeding: A Guide for the Medical Profession:* "Can this infant be safely exposed to this chemical as it appears in breast milk without a risk that exceeds the tremendous benefits of being breast-fed?")

5. Can you monitor the baby for possible symptoms and stop taking the drug in time? If not, can another drug be substituted?

6. If this is a new drug about which little is known, can another, more established drug be substituted?

7. Are you advising me to stop nursing because the maker of the drug does not know what the effects would be or because there are known ill effects?

Among the considerations your doctor will have to weigh are whether this drug is one that can safely be given to a baby of your baby's age, whether the dosage you need will send too much of the drug into your baby's system, and for how long a period you'll need to be taking the drug.

•If it is medically necessary for you to take a certain drug, watch your baby closely for any unusual symptoms—fever, sleepiness, vomiting, unusual crying, loss of appetite, diarrhea, rash, irritability, and so forth. Call her doctor if you notice these or other possible signs of drug effects.

•Take any drug immediately after a feeding so that it will have as much time as possible to work its way through your system before the baby's next nursing.

•If you have to take a medicine that may be harmful to your nursing baby, and if you need to take it for only a short period of time (say, a week or two), you can pump or express your milk during that time and discard it, while feeding your baby formula or previously expressed milk. This way, you'll be keeping up your milk supply and you'll be able to resume nursing as soon as the drug is no longer in your system.

•If you have a question about a certain drug, ask your doctor to consult one of the references listed in this chapter, or to call La Leche League International, 9616 Minneapolis Ave., Franklin Park, IL 60131, (312) 455-7730. A physician on the League's medical advisory board, which keeps abreast of new medications, will tell your doctor what is known about the drug in question.

BIRTH CONTROL PILLS

As we point out in Chapter 9, in our discussion of birth control during lactation, oral contraceptives contain hormones, some of which *may* inhibit the production of milk. While we have no evidence from human studies of their long-term effects on the baby's developing endocrine system, this is a possibility. In most cases, then, it's safest to use a barrier contraceptive during lactation.

DRUGS DURING CHILDBIRTH

Some of the medication given to the mother during labor and delivery passes through the placenta to the baby. The mother's wears off in a few hours, but it may take as much as a week for all the depressant drugs to be eliminated from the baby's immature system. As a result, babies whose mothers received *a great deal* of analgesia and anesthesia during childbirth are likely to be quite sleepy the first few days of life. While this doesn't seem to have a permanent effect on full-size, full-term babies, it does affect their early activities, including their interest in nursing.

Since the vigorous sucking of a hungry baby is vital for establishing an ample supply of milk in the mother, the mother of a sleepy infant who is not interested in nursing is at a definite disadvantage in building up her milk. Pediatrician T. Berry Brazelton compared the breastfeeding responses of babies whose mothers had received average doses of barbiturates two to eight hours before delivery, those who had had an inhalant anesthetic administered during the actual delivery, and those who had received local anesthetics or no medication at all.

The babies of the nonmedicated and locally anesthetized mothers recovered quickly from the ordeal of birth and were nursing and beginning to gain weight by the third day. But the babies of the mothers who had taken barbiturates were not nursing as well and didn't begin to gain weight until the fourth or fifth day. Other research has found that some babies of women who had received local anesthesia are alert but have poor muscle tone that makes it hard for them to nurse.

As in everything else, you need to weigh the relative risks and benefits of various types of pain relief. If, for example, you're in such pain during childbirth that you're worn out and

Drugs That Require a Temporary Cessation of Breastfeeding

It is sometimes necessary for a woman to undergo a diagnostic procedure for which she needs to take a radioactive drug (like Gallium-69, Iodine-125, Iodine-131, or Technetium-99m). If she continued to nurse her baby while the drug was in her system, radioactivity would be present in her milk and would reach her baby. To avoid this, the following steps can be taken:

• Her doctor should consult a nuclear medicine physician who can prescribe the agent with the shortest life in breast milk.

• Breastfeeding should be discontinued for 12 hours to two weeks, depending on the drug. The long-lasting types of these drugs are hardly given any more. Most often, two or three days is the longest one needs to suspend breastfeeding.

• Before the procedure she can pump her breasts and freeze enough milk to feed her baby for the period of time she is not breastfeeding. Or she can buy formula.

• She should continue to pump her breasts (to maintain production) during the time the radioactive agent is present in her body but should discard all of this milk.

overstressed, your ability to nurse will be adversely affected. The best thing, then, is to educate yourself ahead of time about your options, including nonchemical means of pain relief, such as breathing and relaxation techniques, either alone or in combination with lower doses of anesthesia. Many negative effects of drugs are dramatically dose-related, so keeping down the amount you take minimizes the risk.

It's extremely important to discuss with the doctor who'll be assisting in the delivery room the kind of medication that will be prescribed for you while you're in labor. You have to be very clear about what you want, saying, perhaps, something like, "I want to have the least amount of medication possible. I want to avoid general anesthesia. But what if my prepared childbirth techniques are not enough and I'm in a lot of pain? What can I do that will pose the least amount of harm to my baby?" You and your doctor can discuss your situation, in light of your medical history and physical condition, and the two of you can arrive at a possible course of action. The important thing is that you should feel confident that your own needs and those of your baby are carefully considered and that you are getting the best care possible.

Frank W. Summers, M.D., an anesthesiologist in a high-risk obstetric center in California where he attends many complicated births, says, "We are very well aware of the effects of obstetric drugs on labor, delivery, and nursing and we use these drugs with a great deal of thought and care. I want my patients to be as well informed as possible and to be concerned about every part of their medical care. I don't want them panicked, frightened, or guilty if and when anesthetics are used. They should know that the needs of each patient are considered separately at the time the need arises. There are no simple answers."

After you and your doctor have come to an agreement, ask him or her to make a note of the plan on your chart, so that if she or he is not available when you go into labor, whoever is there will be guided by the instructions.

RECREATIONAL AGENTS AND HARD DRUGS

A number of substances that are commonly ingested for non-medical reasons can also have effects on breast milk and breastfed babies. With these, you have more choices about your level of use, or any usage at all.

Tobacco

If you smoke, is breastfeeding still best for your baby? Yes. Would it be better for your baby if you did not smoke, or at least cut down while you're nursing? Again, the answer is yes. Nicotine, the main substance released from cigarettes, passes through your milk to your baby, but most of it is altered in your baby's liver and kidney. Since gastrointestinal absorption is slow, you would expect few if any severe toxic reactions in the nursing baby of a smoking mother. In fact, there is no known evidence of ill effects to any nursing infant.

However, evidence is accumulating about the effects of "passive smoking," that is, inhaling the smoke of other people. Babies are especially vulnerable when the person closest to them is the one breathing smoke on them. (This is true whether a baby is being fed by breast or bottle.) Furthermore, animal experiments have found that nicotine can reduce milk production in laboratory rats, and it's possible that it may also reduce it in humans. It's also possible that the nicotine in the babies' systems may make them fretful. Mothers who stop nursing often do so because they don't have enough milk or because their babies don't seem satisfied. It's good to know that it may be possible to avoid both of these problems simply by not smoking.

If you're pregnant now, you probably know the bad news that smoking causes a wide variety of prenatal complications. (The most conclusive finding relates to the tendency of pregnant smokers to bear smaller babies, and it's harder to establish breastfeeding with a premature or low-birthweight baby.) The good news is that women who stop smoking by the fourth month do not experience these complications.

If you can't stop smoking even for the duration of pregnancy and lactation, or if giving up cigarettes makes you so tense that your milk production is depleted, you can still take some steps that will benefit your baby. You can avoid smoking while you're nursing: Aside from the danger of the tobacco smoke, there's the very real risk of dropping ashes on the baby. You can cut down, smoking as little as possible, especially around your baby. You can make special efforts to smoke in another room or outdoors. And you can smoke immediately after a feeding rather than shortly before one.

Alcohol

Alcohol in moderation is a relaxant; in excess it acts as a depressant. There's no evidence that moderate amounts of alcohol—a couple of glasses of beer or wine, or a cocktail or two in one day—will have any ill effects on your nursing baby. In fact, they may even help to supply more milk by helping

Drugs That Should Not Be Taken by Nursing Mothers

DRUG	REASON
Amethopterin	May suppress baby's immune system. Has unknown effect on growth or association with cancer.
Bromocriptine (Parlodel)	Inhibits prolactin secretion, decreases milk supply.
Chemotherapeutic agents	These drugs are given precisely because they kill cells in the body. There is a danger, therefore, that even a tiny dose may have harmful effects on the cells in the baby's system.
Cimetidine (Tagamet, Peptol)	May suppress baby's gastric acidity, inhibit ability to metabolize drugs, and unduly stimulate the central nervous system.
Clemastine (Tavist)	Causes drowsiness, irritability, refusal to eat, high-pitched cry, and neck stiffness.

you to relax. For most women the early evening feeding is usually the scantiest of the day due to maternal fatigue and the stresses of the day. An occasional mild drink before dinner (yours and your baby's) may be able to stimulate your let-down reflex.

Heavy drinking, however, is another story altogether. It can affect your ability to care for your baby, and it can make your nursing baby drowsy by depressing the nervous system.

The jury is still out about *any* drinking during pregnancy. While some health professionals believe that an occasional

Cyclophosphamide (Cytoxan, Neosar, Procytox)	May suppress baby's immune system. Has unknown effect on growth or association with cancer.
Ergotamine (Ergomar, Ergostat, Gynergen, Wigrettes)	Doses used in medicines for migraine headaches can cause vomiting, diarrhea, and convulsions in baby. May decrease milk supply.
Gold salts (Myochrysine)	Can cause rash, and inflammation of kidney and liver.
Iodine (sometimes found in cough syrup)	Can affect thyroid function.
Methimazole (Tapazole)	May interfere with thyroid function.
Phenindione	Can cause hemorrhage.
Thiouracil	Can affect thyroid function. (This does not apply to propylthiouracil.)
Tetracycline (Achromycin, Cefracycline, Novatetra, Sumycin)	Can discolor and interfere with calcification of developing teeth of baby if used for more than 10 days.

social drink is not harmful, others advise pregnant women not to drink alcohol for the entire nine months.

Marijuana

We know less about marijuana than about any other intoxicant. We do know that its most active ingredient is fat-soluble and does appear in breast milk. It's also capable of being stored in the body for a long time, even after a single exposure. Since studies of nursing animals have shown structural changes in brain cells and drowsiness in nursing pups after their mothers were exposed to marijuana, it certainly seems prudent for pregnant and nursing women to abstain from it.

Cocaine

So far there is nothing in the medical literature about the effects of cocaine on breastfeeding. This is, however, a powerful and dangerous drug, which goes through the milk and which carries the risk of overstimulating the nervous system of the nursing baby of a cocaine-using mother (causing irritability and difficulty in sleeping). Pregnant and nursing women should not use it at all in any form, and women who cannot abstain should stop breastfeeding for their baby's sake and enroll in a treatment program for their own sake.

Recent reports have described serious behavioral and health problems in babies born to women who used cocaine during pregnancy, which underscores the dangers inherent in this drug. Many people underestimate the risks, convinced that its occasional use at a party will do little harm. First, cocaine can be fatal—even in a small dosage, regardless of your previous drug history. Second, many people who began as social users have become addicted. It seems plain that anyone using cocaine is playing with fire and that a pregnant or nursing woman risks injuring her baby in the flames.

Amphetamines

Again, while there's nothing in the literature about the effects of this drug on nursing infants, these are powerful stimulants that can overstimulate a baby's nervous system. Therefore, they should be avoided by both pregnant and nursing women.

Barbiturates

While these drugs can apparently be taken safely by nursing mothers in the usual small medical doses, overuse of them can be dangerous to both mother and baby. For the user they can be addictive or even fatal. They are particularly dangerous when they are taken with alcohol, and nearly one third of accidental drug-related deaths are related to barbiturate overdose. If a mother takes enough barbiturates to put her to sleep, the baby may be adversely affected. Again, this is a class of drugs to stay away from, especially when you are nursing.

Heroin

Women addicted to heroin are more likely to bear premature babies who have become addicted to the drug within the womb. If a mother is in a detoxification program after the birth, continuing to breastfeed will help her baby rid its system of the drug, as well. If she is going to continue to use heroin, however, breastfeeding can be dangerous to the baby. The heroin does go through the milk and may affect the baby even more than it does the mother.

A nursing mother has many choices to make. Her decision about the substances to which she will expose both herself and her baby is one of the most important, both during pregnancy and when she and the baby become a nursing couple. Now let's talk about the actual launching of the breastfeeding journey, as you and your baby become a nursing couple.

7

Starting
Out Right

Finally you set eyes upon that squalling, squirming mite of humanity whose arrival you have so eagerly awaited all these months. You marvel at the wonder of tiny fingers and toes. You are amazed to realize that this small person actually grew in your body. You draw the little body close to you, to cuddle and love.

And then questions rush through your mind. How will you be able to care for such a dependent little creature? How will you know what to do? And when and how to do it? It may buoy up your confidence to stop for a minute and consider that women have been having first babies for millions of years and have somehow coped well enough so that each succeeding generation has survived to bear its own progeny.

Like every other new mother, you have questions about every aspect of child care—how to diaper, burp, bathe and dress your baby. Probably your biggest concern revolves around feeding your baby. In this chapter we talk about the first few days after birth, when you and your baby take your first steps toward becoming a nursing couple.

The first two weeks constitute a time when you and your baby need to learn about each other and about breastfeeding. Human beings do not have instincts; we have to *learn* how to nurse our babies. (Actually, other animals do, too. Not long ago, when the San Diego Zoo was troubled because its gorilla was not nursing her infant, the zoo asked some local nursing women to go and take seats in front of the gorilla's cage so that she could learn from their example!)

If you know what to expect and what to do, you'll be better prepared for these first few weeks. You can make the beginning of breastfeeding easier if you arm yourself with information, if you start out right, and if you know where to go for help. Meanwhile, you may need to be patient to give the two of you time to develop your relationship as a nursing couple. You may have a love-at-first-sight relationship, with nothing but good experiences right from the start. Or you may have a longer courtship, not establishing a smooth and mutually satisfying bond for a couple of months. Either way, if your experience is like most other women's, breastfeeding will get better and better for both you and your baby.

BREASTFEEDING IN HOSPITAL OR BIRTHING CENTER

The growth of modern hospitals as places for babies to be born coincided with the popularity of feeding those babies with bottles of formula. So it's not surprising that many hospital routines were developed to fit the patterns of bottle-fed babies—and the convenience of hospital staff. Some of these routines include separating mother and baby, feeding infants on strict four-hour schedules, and limiting the length of feeding sessions.

In recent years, however, many hospital administrators have changed their routines in the recognition that breastfed babies thrive best on a very different schedule. As this has been happening, it's become apparent that many of the changes fought for by nursing mothers and by those who care for them have been better for the physical and emotional health of bottle-fed babies, too.

THE IDEAL BEGINNING

In the best of all possible worlds, every baby would be born healthy, after the full gestation period. Every mother would have an easy, fast, unmedicated delivery. Both mother and baby would be alert and feeling good. Right after birth the mother would put her baby to the breast. The baby would latch on and nurse eagerly. Mother and baby would then spend their time together, in the same room, where the mother would rest, nursing the baby every time he wanted to feed. She would have supportive health care professionals to go to with her questions, as well as helpful friends and relatives.

In the real world, this scenario *sometimes* unfolds exactly as it's written here. Most often, however, one or more of the elements just described are not present. Some babies are born prematurely; some mothers have long, difficult deliveries or cesarean sections for which they need some form of anesthesia; some hospitals do not permit immediate breastfeeding, demand feeding, or rooming-in; some babies are not eager nursers. And still mothers and babies can and do go on to have wonderful breastfeeding experiences. Let's look at how much you can do to achieve this scenario—and what you can do when you need to follow a different script.

Healthy Mother, Healthy Baby

Getting good prenatal care and taking good care of yourself and your unborn child throughout your pregnancy are the best things you can do toward improving your chances for bearing a healthy, full-term baby. Preparing yourself for childbirth will improve your chances for a drug-free delivery and, as a result, a wide-awake baby. If, however, unforeseen circumstances occur and your baby's birth turns out differently from the way you planned it, don't berate yourself. Instead, focus on what you can do now for your baby and yourself. We'll talk specifically about postcesarean breastfeeding later in this chapter and in Chapter 13 we'll talk about nursing premature babies.

Breastfeeding Within One Hour of Childbirth

Recent research has confirmed the value of doing what most mothers intuitively want to do—nurse their babies as soon as they're born. Babies fed within one hour of birth pass their first stool earlier and have lower levels of *bilirubin* (a waste product formed by the breaking down of red blood cells; high levels in the blood cause jaundice, which we'll talk about in Chapter 13).

Even though the true milk has not yet come into your breasts, they have, from the last weeks of pregnancy, had a rich supply of colostrum, that sweet yellowish fluid that provides such a good start to an infant's life. (See Chapter 3.) While your baby is getting the benefits of colostrum, she is also helping to establish her future food supply. The best way to produce an abundance of milk is to allow a hungry infant to suck vigorously and frequently soon after birth. The more she sucks, the more milk you will produce.

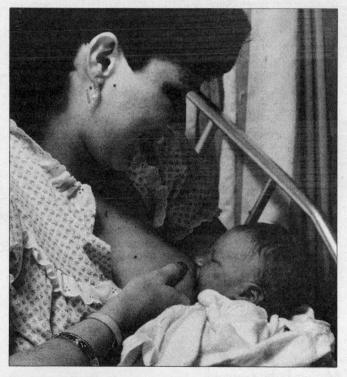

Some newborns, like this one, are eager nursers right from the start; others need a little time to get going.

As in so many cases, the most natural thing is the best thing. For you, the most natural time to offer your breast to your baby will be as soon after birth as possible. The exact time for this will vary, depending largely on how you are feeling, how your baby is doing, and where you give birth.

If you were awake during your delivery in a facility that encourages natural childbirth, you may be permitted to hold and nurse your baby moments after he emerges from your body. This is ideal, since the baby is likely to be more wide awake now than he will be several hours later. Since stimulation of the breasts causes the uterus to contract, the baby's immediate suckling can speed delivery of the placenta. The contractions of the uterus also shut off the maternal blood vessels that formerly fed the baby and, thus, help to discourage excessive bleeding.

In some hospitals, however, the mother may glimpse or hold her baby momentarily after birth but will not be permitted to breastfeed for several hours. Doctors sometimes justify this delay by their concern that the baby may not be able to swallow properly and may get into serious trouble by taking food into the windpipe. For this reason they may hold off breastfeeding until after the baby has had a bottle or two of water, showing normal swallowing function. None of this is necessary, however—neither the delay nor the water. Colostrum is easily absorbed and nonirritating, and giving a newborn anything in a bottle can cause "nipple confusion," which we'll talk more about shortly.

Immediate breastfeeding is not a good idea if you are very drowsy from heavy medication or if your baby is very premature, tiny, or fragile. If you cannot nurse right away, either because of hospital regulations, your condition, or your baby's, don't worry. Immediate is best, but later is not disastrous.

Immediate breastfeeding is one of those issues that you should discuss with your doctor and hospital before you give birth, letting everyone involved know that you want to do this, and asking your doctor to leave orders accordingly.

Mother-Baby Contact

All other things being equal, mothers and babies usually do best when they're close to each other. This is easy to achieve

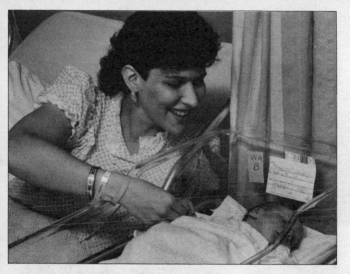

*With rooming-in, mother and baby can get
acquainted sooner and can nurse on demand.*

at a birthing center or at home, and in those hospitals that
have rooming-in. This policy lets you keep your baby in your
own room rather than in the newborn nursery, either around
the clock or during daytime hours only. It's comforting for
both partners and it provides a get-acquainted opportunity for
both you and your husband to get to know your baby and learn
her natural eating and sleeping rhythms.

Being together makes the beginning of breastfeeding that
much easier, since you can nurse your baby when she's hungry
and awake, without having to depend on her being brought to
you on a set schedule or when it's convenient for the nurse in
the newborn nursery. Only through living with your baby can
you adjust your milk supply to her needs.

Again, this is one of those issues you will have thought
about before birth, one that will have entered into your decision about where to have your baby.

All other things are not always equal, of course. If you're
exhausted from a hard labor and delivery you may not feel up
to caring for your baby all day long. If your baby needs special

care, he may have to be in another room. So you may not be together for the first few days of your baby's life, but you will, of course, be "rooming in" as soon as you get home. If you don't have rooming-in, ask to have your baby brought to you as soon as possible after he awakens in the nursery.

Your baby should not be receiving any bottles in the hospital. While some babies are adaptable enough to go back and forth between bottle and breast with hardly a break in rhythm, others become confused when they're asked to alternate between suckling at the breast and drinking from a rubber nip-

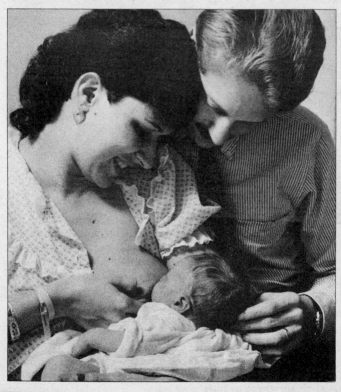

The father is an important member of the nursing family right from the start.

ple. As we pointed out in Chapter 1, the two forms of feeding require different mouth movements. Furthermore, since milk flows more easily from the rubber nipple, babies fed bottles early in their lives sometimes get used to this and are less willing to expend the effort required for nursing. This "nipple confusion" can lead to sucking problems, so it's best to avoid the possibility if you can.

Don't worry, though, if you can't be with your baby for the first two or three days after birth. You'll have plenty of time to make up for it afterward. Many mothers and babies have had limited contact at first and still gone on to forge strong breastfeeding relationships.

A great deal has been written about the parent-child "bonding" that is said to take place immediately after birth. In the mid-1970s, some pediatric researchers maintained that the first few hours after birth were critical for a deep attachment to take place and that if mother and baby were separated during this time, bonding would not occur and the emotional ramifications of its absence could last for years.

After subsequent research failed, however, to find long-term effects of early contact, the original spokesmen for the theory modified their position to say that this early contact was not essential for strong bonding to take place. So if you and your baby are not together right after the birth, don't let your disappointment at missing this special, intimate time turn into unnecessary worry and guilt over your baby's future development. Human beings are remarkably resilient, and babies can overcome the most traumatic early experiences to grow up to be healthy and well-adjusted.

Hospital Help

If your doctor, midwife, and/or nurses are knowledgeable and supportive of breastfeeding, don't hesitate to take your questions to them. They have probably heard most of them before and will be able to advise and reassure you. Ask whether you can call on them with questions after you go home with your baby; chances are they'll be happy to continue to help. If you're in a rarer situation these days and your doctor or nurses give lip service to breastfeeding without providing real help, or they act as if they don't want to be bothered, or they want to help but give contradictory advice, you'll have to get your help from other sources. (See "Developing Your Support Network" in Chapter 4.)

Speak Up in the Hospital

•Ask your doctor to leave written orders for hospital personnel at the time of your baby's delivery, specifying the following: You are not to receive any drugs to dry up your milk; your baby is not to receive any bottles of formula or water (you may want to pin a note to this effect on the baby's nightgown or blanket); your baby is to be brought to you on demand or at least every three hours around the clock.

•Communicate the information yourself to the nursery staff when you first go into the hospital. Remind your baby's doctor and any nurses who come to you that you are planning to breastfeed and that you should not receive any drugs to dry up your milk. (If you have received some, don't worry. Putting your baby to the breast will still bring in your milk.)

•Remind your doctor and nurses that you want to feed your baby during the night, as well as during the day. Your breasts need the stimulation, and your baby needs your milk.

•If you are modest about breastfeeding in front of your roommate, pull the curtain around your bed. If necessary, ask for help.

•If you need help positioning your baby at the breast, ask the nursery nurse to help you.

•If your breasts are filling up uncomfortably between feedings, ask the nurse to help you hand-express some of your milk or ask whether the hospital has an electric breast pump that you can use to pump just enough to relieve the fullness. (See the Appendix.)

•If you're uncomfortable for any reason at all, tell your doctor and nurse.

•If you have any questions at all, ask them. The only dumb question is the one you *don't* ask.

You can do a great deal to help yourself in the hospital. Most important, you need to be informed and assertive. You are only one patient among many. Hospital personnel have other things on their minds, and they may not be as closely attuned to your wishes as you would like. Don't be shy about asking or reminding them about aspects of care that are important for you and your baby. If you're polite and pleasant, no one is likely to take offense. Some of the points you may want to bring up are listed in the box on page 124 (Speak Up in the Hospital).

Suppose you meet with resistance in every quarter. Or you're in a nonsupportive hospital with outdated regulations (such as four-hour feeding schedules and feeding nursing babies bottles of water). If you have a full-term, healthy baby and someone to help you at home, it may be possible and advisable for you to leave the hospital within 12 to 24 hours of giving birth. Even if you have to stay the full time (usually only three days) in a less than ideal setting, take heart. You'll be within these walls only a short time. Many other women have borne babies in much more restrictive circumstances and have gone on to nurse them successfully. You can, too.

BRINGING THE BABY TO THE BREAST

Every new mother feels awkward the first few times she puts her baby to her breast. You have to learn an entire new set of movements and sensations. No matter how much you've read or how many other nursing babies you've seen, it's very different when you're actually doing it yourself. Just like riding a bicycle. So be patient at the beginning and be reassured that before long you'll both become experts. And—again like riding a bicycle—once you learn, you never forget.

Whether your baby first comes to you right after birth or several hours later, he may not at first show a great interest in nursing. Many babies do not nurse well at all for their first few days. One study of 600 newborns found that 40 percent of them had to be actively helped to suck. They have to learn what it's all about, too. Some babies start out by licking their mothers' nipples, which is a fine get-acquainted maneuver and also serves the practical function of making the nipples erect. Eventually, with the help you give them, their inborn reflexes assert themselves and they begin to nurse.

If your baby is sleepy the first couple of times, offer your breast and try to rouse him by using the techniques listed in the box below (Waking a Sleepy Baby). Even if none of these techniques work at first, don't worry about it. He may suck in his sleep or he may enjoy the experience so much that he decides it's worth waking up for. Even if he sleeps through his first meal or two, he'll wake up when he's ready.

Waking a Sleepy Baby

The following suggestions will sometimes rouse a sleepy baby enough to interest him in nursing.

• If the room isn't too cold, take off all clothing but the diaper. The feel of the air may do the trick.

• Sit the baby on your lap and lean him forward slightly—not to an extreme jack-knifed position, which can cause damage to his spleen. Then walk your fingers up the back of his spine.

• Gently massage his legs and arms.

• Give him a sponge bath.

• Dab him on the forehead with a sponge dampened with cool water.

• Express a little milk into his mouth.

Normal full-term infants are born with enough reserves to keep them healthy even if they go without eating anything for two or three days. Aside from the healthy colostrum they receive, the first few feeding sessions are more for education—yours and the baby's—than for nourishment. (These early nursings are sometimes called "practice feeds.")

During the first couple of days, while your milk supply is becoming established, you learn how to nurse and your baby learns how to suckle. Of course, it's easier for both parties if your baby is an eager pupil. But if not—if she keeps yawning or snoozing, or can't get the nipple in her mouth or keeps letting go of it—don't worry. She'll make up for it. Meanwhile, you can use these first few visits for such important activities as feeling downy-soft hair, inspecting tiny fingers and toes, and getting used to the feeling of being a mother.

Finding a Comfortable Position for Nursing

It's worth taking the time and the effort to find good positions for nursing. One of the most exciting findings of recent years is the importance of good positioning for good suckling. Kittie Frantz, R.N., director of the Breastfeeding Infant Clinic, Los Angeles County, and her colleagues at the University of Southern California Medical Center found that many cases of women with sore nipples and babies who failed to gain weight could be traced to poor positioning at the breast. By readjust-

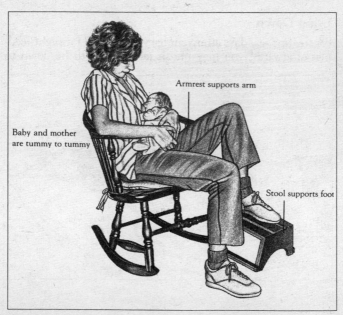

Nursing while sitting up.

ing nursing positions, both of these problems were often cleared up.

When you find two or three comfortable positions, alternate them. This will help to prevent sore nipples by spreading out the pressure on different parts of your breast. It will also serve to stimulate different milk ducts, and thus to prevent clogged ducts.

A good nursing position should incorporate the following:

• You are supported in such a way that you can hold the position for some time without feeling cramped or stiff; you are not hunched over, trying to bring the breast to your baby; instead, you bring the baby to the breast.

• Your baby's body is face-to-face with yours; her mouth is directly facing the nipple; she is close enough to take much or all of the areola into her mouth while nursing.

Lying Down

For the first few days after your baby's birth and for night feedings afterwards, you may find it most restful to lie down to

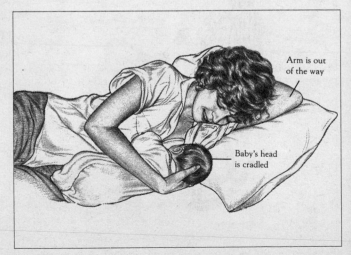

Nursing while lying down.

nurse. Or you may feel more comfortable sitting up for every feeding.

To nurse lying down, lie on your side with one or two pillows behind your back and one or two under your head. A flat pillow (made of folded cloth diapers, a receiving blanket, or a towel) placed under the baby's head as he lies facing you will put his mouth at breast level and make it easier for him to reach the nipple. Your bottom arm can be up and out of the way of his head, or under the baby's head, cradling him.

If you had a cesarean birth, ask your nurse to make you comfortable. Being a good patient means getting well and taking good care of your baby; it does not mean "not bothering the nurses." They want to help you. Keep your legs bent, with a pillow between your knees. Ask the nurse to place something firm at the bottom of your bed to push your feet against.

There are two ways to shift position from nursing on one side to the other. One is to nurse the baby on the bottom breast, then to tuck that breast under your bottom arm and to lean over the baby and nurse with the top breast. At the next feeding you switch sides. The other way of changing involves nursing on one side, then pulling the baby over onto your stomach and rolling both you and your baby over to your other side, using the guard-rail on the side of the bed to help. Ask the nurse to show you how.

Sitting Up

Sit straight up in bed or in a comfortable chair or couch, with your back and head supported by one or more big pillows if necessary. Put the baby on a pillow on your lap if necessary in order to bring her mouth to nipple level. Raise one or both knees to bring her closer to your body. It may help to support your foot on the side the baby's nursing from by resting it on a chair rung, a footstool, or a large book.

The baby should be lying on her side so that she does not have to turn her head to reach the nipple. The baby's face, abdomen, genitals, and knees should all be facing your body. Her pelvis should be up against your abdomen. The baby's lower arm is under your arm and around your waist, pinned out of her way. Your arm on the side of the breast she's nursing from supports her head as you hold her in the crook of your

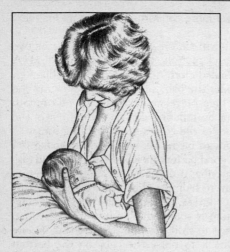

The "football hold" is especially good for twins, cesarean mothers, and babies who need special help with sucking technique.

elbow. Your arm is extended as far down the baby's back as possible, with your hand holding her buttocks or upper thigh, keeping her as close to your body as you can. Her knees are held across your other breast, not hanging down. She is horizontal, not diagonal.

An alternate position is the "football hold." In this position you tuck the baby under your arm like a football. His head rests on a pillow on your lap; his feet are behind your back. This position is good for cesarean mothers, since the baby's legs cannot kick or put pressure on the incision. It's also good for twins. And some babies who don't suck properly in the other positions do fine this way.

Latching On

When you and your baby are in position, you're ready to "plug him in," as one five-year-old said of his baby brother. Many babies find the nipple easily, latch onto the breast right away, and take off as if they were born knowing what to do. (Apparently they were.) Others need to learn how. If your baby seems to need help, this is what you can do:

Support your breast with your free hand. Your fingers should not touch the areola. (If they do, they will be in the baby's way, preventing him from taking it into his mouth properly.) Your thumb should be on top of your breast, your fingers below it. Do not use the "cigarette" hold, in which your index finger is on top of the areola, since this sometimes interferes with a baby's grasp of the nipple.

Moving your breast with your hand, tease your baby's mouth open by tickling his lips with your nipple. Lightly touch his lips, going from upper to lower and back again. When the baby opens his mouth wide (like a yawn), quickly draw his body close to you and center your breast in his mouth. Let him grab for it; don't just stuff it in his mouth. If he does not open his mouth wide at first, repeat the tickling procedure and wait until he does before you put your breast in his mouth.

Another way to draw a baby to the breast is to hold him against you so that a corner of his mouth touches your nipple or to stroke one of his cheeks with the nipple until he turns his mouth to it. This capitalizes on his inborn "rooting reflex." When he opens his mouth, gently bring him closer. If his legs curve closely around your body, his body will be at the correct angle.

Do not try to open the baby's mouth by pressing in on both cheeks. The natural tendency is to turn toward the side

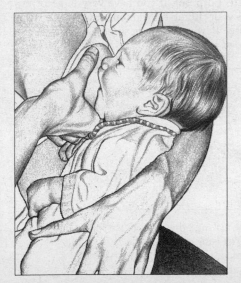

It helps a baby latch on if the mother supports her breast with her free hand— especially if she has large breasts.

being touched; if both are touched at once, babies become confused and move their mouths frantically from side to side. Do not push his head onto the breast. He may become frightened as his nose is pushed into your flesh and be more likely to wail his frustration than to seize the opportunity to nurse.

When properly positioned, the baby's jaws will go beyond the nipple to come together on the areola, about an inch and a half in, not on the nipple itself. This is very important for the prevention of sore nipples.

If your baby takes only the nipple into her mouth, take her off the breast and start over again. If you let her mouth the nipple alone, she won't be able to get any milk and you'll get sore nipples. It is important for her to take enough of the areola into her mouth to enable her to "gum" or "jaw" the breast. It is the up-and-down pressure of the infant's jaws that makes the ducts under the areola release the milk.

If your baby pushes your breast out with her tongue, take the breast away and start over again. Keep doing this until she gets it right.

Her nose should be touching the breast. If she's facing you squarely, she will be able to breathe. Babies' noses are very flat (probably for just this purpose). If you have very large or engorged breasts, press your thumb on your breast to keep it away from the baby's nose. If your breast is so engorged that the baby cannot get a good grip, express a little bit of milk by hand

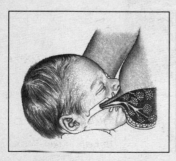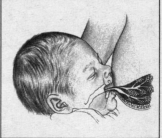

The baby on the left is sucking correctly, with the entire areola in her mouth. The baby on the right, who is sucking only on the nipple, should be gently taken off the breast and put back again until she is nursing correctly.

and then bring her back to the breast. (For suggestions on relieving engorgement, see Chapter 12.) Be sure that she can breathe through her nose, since most babies won't open their mouths to breathe unless they're forced to. (This is why babies are so distressed when they catch a cold.)

Feeling the Let-Down Reflex

Within minutes after you begin to nurse, you may feel a tingling "pins-and-needles" sensation. It may appear within the first minute of nursing, not for several minutes, or not at all. Most women feel this sign of the *let-down reflex*, also known as the *milk-ejection reflex*. Some, however, who produce a lot of milk, do not.

Whether felt or not, the let-down marks the passage of milk from your breast. You may be aware of milk dripping or spurting from the other breast, or you may not. Eventually you'll experience let-down at various times throughout the day, sometimes when you just think about your baby.

You may also feel "after-pains," abdominal pains similar to menstrual cramps. They may be very mild or surprisingly strong. The pains are apt to be stronger for women who have borne children before. Be happy when you feel them, because they tell you that your uterus is contracting and that your let-down reflex is operating. If you're really uncomfortable, your doctor may prescribe a mild pain reliever. In any case, these pains are short-lived; though your uterus will continue to shrink for about six weeks, you'll be aware of the contractions only for the first few days after childbirth.

Taking the Baby Off the Breast

When it's time for the baby to stop nursing, insert your finger in the side of his mouth to break the suction between his mouth and your breast. Do not try to pull him off the nipple. He will automatically tighten his mouth, which can be quite painful and can contribute to sore nipples.

One Breast or Two?

Try to offer both breasts at each feeding. This will give your baby more milk, will stimulate your production of milk, and will help to prevent engorgement. Don't take the baby away from the first breast while she's actively nursing. Wait until she stops to rest; then make the change. If she falls asleep on the first breast, changing her diaper and/or burping her may wake her up enough to interest her in the second breast. If not, you can express milk from the second breast and save it for a future feeding.

Since the first breast is usually emptied more completely, alternate first choice at each feeding, starting on the side that was suckled last at the previous feeding. To keep track of first and second servings, pin a safety pin to your bra on the side that was offered first; switch the pin at every feeding. Or you can switch a ring, bracelet, or rubber band from hand to hand or stick a little square of surgical tape on your chest above the just suckled breast. (The tape shouldn't hurt, especially if you change its location from time to time.)

HOW FREQUENTLY SHOULD YOU NURSE YOUR NEW BABY?

In many societies around the world, mothers and their nursing infants are constantly together, and mothers nurse their babies every time the baby fidgets, squirms, or makes a sound. Among the !Kung people, who live in the Kalahari Desert in Botswana, babies nurse on demand several times an hour, day and night. This may involve 48 feedings in one day! Not surprisingly, the babies gain well.

In our society women are often cautioned not to feed their babies too frequently as a way of protecting their nipples. (!Kung women would be surprised to hear this, since they don't develop sore nipples.) Many hospitals still keep babies on a four-hour schedule, which may suit the needs of formula-fed babies, but which is totally unsuitable for the breastfed. Even the more progressive three-hour schedule may not be frequent enough in the early days of a baby's life.

At the beginning it's better for both of you to nurse for short periods quite often during the day (and night) than to space the feedings farther apart and to nurse longer at each feeding. Recent research indicates that mothers and babies do

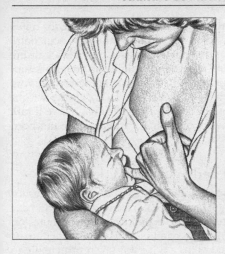

Taking the baby off the breast is easy and painless if you break the suction by inserting your finger in the side of his mouth.

best when nursings average between 10 and 12 times a day during the first couple of weeks (an average of every two hours). One study found that mothers who fed their new babies 10 times a day nursed a total of 138 minutes in a 24-hour period, compared to mothers who nursed seven times a day for a total of 137 minutes. Even though total time of nursing was almost identical, the more frequently nursed babies had a much larger weight gain than the other babies. This is not surprising, since, as we saw in Chapter 3, the baby's stimulation of the mother's nipples causes her prolactin levels to rise and the higher her prolactin, the more milk she produces. Babies nurse more vigorously at the beginning of a feeding, stimulating the breasts to a greater degree. Other research confirms that more frequent nursings result in a more bounteous milk supply and greater gains in babies' lengths and weights.

Your milk will come in sooner if you begin to nurse early and then nurse frequently. Women who do this usually get their milk on the second day after birth, while those who begin to nurse later and keep to four-hour schedules don't get theirs till the third day, or later. Frequent nursings carry another benefit, too. Newborn babies who are nursed often are less likely to become jaundiced. For a more complete discussion of jaundice, turn to Chapter 12.

More important than counting feedings per day or hours between feedings, however, is paying attention to your baby. When he cries, it's appropriate to nurse him. He's gaining good practice in nursing and you're building up your milk supply. He's being comforted and you're not going crazy trying to figure out a way to stop his crying. He's gaining weight and you're gaining confidence. In the next chapter we'll talk more about the way demand feeding works *after* the newborn period.

How Long Should Early Nursing Periods Last?

Doctors used to advise new mothers to nurse their babies for only one minute on each breast at each feeding for the first day of nursing; two minutes on the second day; three minutes on the third; and so on until a maximum of 10 minutes per breast per feeding was reached. This advice was given principally to prevent sore nipples. The only trouble was that it didn't work. Many women still got sore nipples, but they felt the tenderness two or three days later than they would have otherwise. (For ways to treat sore nipples, see Chapter 12.)

The big problem with such short nursing periods is that they don't give the let-down reflex a chance to work. It often takes several minutes of nursing for the let-down reflex of a new mother to take effect. Furthermore, if nipple discomfort occurs, it's most apt to appear when the baby is first latching on to the breast. Taking the baby from the breast before the milk lets down is frustrating for the baby who doesn't get the milk and for the mother who is left with her breasts full of milk, a situation that can lead to painful engorgement, clogged ducts, or infection.

A more realistic nursing schedule that works well for many new mothers involves letting the baby suckle for five minutes at each breast at each feeding for the first day (some newborns, however, won't be ready to stay at the breast this long); 10 minutes for the second; and 15 minutes or as long as the baby wants to thereafter. One study of 2,000 babies aged two to three weeks found that their feeding sessions lasted from 10 to 60 minutes, averaging half an hour.

Instead of watching the clock, however, it's better to watch your baby. You can tell when a baby is actively nursing.

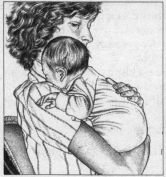
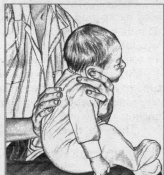
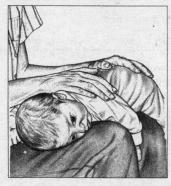

These illustrations show the three best ways to effectively burp your baby. Babies feel much better when they burp up bubbles of air after feedings. Amazingly loud burps sometimes erupt from the mouths of tiny infants.

You can hear her swallowing; you can see her jaws and temples working, you can see her cheeks being sucked in. When she stops suckling, take her off the breast. If she falls asleep at the breast, burp her after one breast and put her to the other. In the next chapter we'll talk more about nursing sessions after the newborn period and about how to tell whether your baby is getting enough to eat.

Burping the Baby

Sometimes babies swallow air during a feeding. If they can bring this up in the form of a hearty burp, they'll be more comfortable and ready to nurse some more. Breastfed babies usually swallow less air than do bottle-fed infants, and some nurslings hardly ever burp after a feeding. Others invariably do, especially if you produce a great deal of milk so that your baby has to gulp to keep up with the supply. Babies often spit up milk when they burp. This is normal. (If your baby vomits forcefully, so that the milk spurts vigorously out of his mouth for some distance, call your doctor.)

After your baby has finished suckling from one breast, it's time to burp him. You can then diaper him, put him to the other breast, and then let him drift off to sleep as he finishes nursing.

There are three effective burping positions:

•Hold him vertically with his head over your shoulder.

•Sit him on your lap, supporting his head with one hand.

•Lay him on his stomach across your knees.

Put a diaper in front of the baby's face to catch any spit-up milk and then gently rub or pat his back. Don't pound him hard! He won't like it and he won't bring up his burps any faster. If he hasn't burped in a few minutes, don't worry about it. Go ahead and give him the other breast. When he has finished nursing, lay him down on his stomach or his side, so that he'll be able to bring up any air that's still in his stomach.

BOWEL MOVEMENTS

While your baby was still cradled in your womb, her bodily organs started to function. At about the sixth month of fetal life, a mass of cast-off cells from her liver, pancreas, and gall bladder began to form in her intestines, remaining there until birth. This dark green tarlike substance called *meconium* is excreted in her bowel movements during the first couple of days after birth. Its elimination seems to be speeded up by the colostrum she gets from your breasts.

Once the meconium is out of your baby's system, her stools will range in color from a golden daffodil yellow to a yellow-green to a brownish tint. The bowel movements of a breastfed baby are usually looser and more frequent than those of a formula-fed baby. They're milder-smelling, too.

When you're changing your baby daughter's diapers a few days after birth, you may notice some bleeding from the vagina. This "false menstruation" is due to hormones secreted by the placenta just before birth. It will stop in a day or two and is nothing to worry about.

WEIGHT LOSS AFTER BIRTH

All newborn babies lose weight after birth, mostly because of their elimination of birth fluids and meconium. A loss of up to 10 percent of birth weight is common, although some healthy babies lose even more than that. We used to believe that breastfed babies regained birth weight more slowly than bottle-fed babies, but this now seems to be more a result of restricting nursings, making them too short and too far apart. Your baby will gain weight faster if you nurse frequently.

Do not weigh your baby yourself. You'll only make yourself anxious for no good reason. Most home baby scales are not accurate and don't reflect either the amount of milk a baby is taking or the amount of weight gained from day to day. In the next chapter we'll talk about ways to tell whether your baby seems to be gaining weight, and you'll get confirmation of her progress when you take her to the doctor for her examination at one month of age.

NEWBORN HEALTH MEASURES

Immediately after birth your baby should receive vitamin K, which is essential for helping his blood to clot and for preventing hemorrhagic disease of the newborn. While the intestines will produce vitamin K within a few days of birth, infants are born without it. This vitamin is present at insufficiently low levels in breast milk, and thus breastfed babies need to have it administered separately. Bottle-fed babies receive it in their formula.

Within one hour of birth your baby should also receive special eye drops if there is any chance at all that you might have or be a carrier of gonorrhea. If the baby was born in a hospital or birthing center, both vitamin K and eye drops will be administered by the obstetric staff. If she was born at home, your birth attendant should have taken care of these important preventive health measures.

A few days after birth your baby should be tested to be sure that he does not suffer from one of several rare birth disorders that can now be easily identified and treated. These screening tests can be performed on a single sample of a few drops of the baby's blood. If your baby is born in a hospital, you'll be informed of the procedures, which can be performed there within two weeks of birth. If you have your baby elsewhere or if you leave the hospital the same day, you can find out how to have this screening performed by calling your local department of health.

When these tests were first administered, some hospitals required all newborns to receive one or more bottles of formula for the purpose of the testing. We now know that it is not necessary to give your breastfed baby formula for this purpose.

CESAREAN BIRTH

If your baby was born by cesarean section, your breasts filled up with milk just as soon as if you had given birth vaginally. There is no reason at all why you cannot breastfeed successfully. You may begin to breastfeed a few hours or a day later, depending on how you feel, but the sooner you begin, the better you're likely to feel and the faster you'll recover from your surgery.

Be sure to tell your doctor ahead of time, as well as the hospital anesthesiologist, that you plan to breastfeed your baby, and that you want medication and treatment compatible with your baby's well-being, as well as your own. After the surgery, it's okay to get relief from your pain through narcotics, which may be administered by injection or pills. The American Academy of Pediatrics has gone on record to state that the benefits of breastfeeding outweigh the negative consequences of a baby's being slightly sleepy from such medication. You don't have to suffer to breastfeed!

You'll probably stay in the hospital a couple of days longer than women who deliver vaginally. And you'll need more rest, both in the hospital and at home. Because of your abdominal incision, you'll want to make special efforts to find comfort-

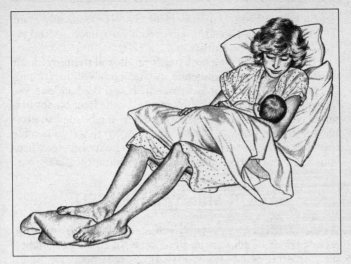

Mothers who have delivered their babies by cesarean birth appreciate lots of pillows. If your hospital can't supply them, have someone bring them from home.

able positions for breastfeeding. Ask the hospital nurses for help and experiment with different positions until you find the one that you like best. You'll need to position your baby so she isn't lying across or kicking the site of your incision. The most popular postcesarean nursing positions are: sitting up, with pillows on the mother's lap to bring the baby up to breast level; the football hold; and lying down.

A GIFT THAT YOU DON'T WANT

Many hospitals present each new mother with a free six-pack of formula when she leaves the hospital with her baby, even if she is breastfeeding. This often has more to do with aggressive promotion practices of the formula manufacturers than with the belief that this is important. A number of hospitals have discontinued this practice and have found that breastfeeding rates have risen accordingly. In fact, the new guidelines from

the New York State Department of Health specifically man-
date that formula should be given out only upon special re-
quest by a doctor or mother.

If your hospital offers you free formula, tell them you don't
want it. Show your confidence in your body's ability to produce the milk that your baby needs. If you do decide to use
formula for an occasional supplemental bottle later on, it's better to buy it then after your own milk is established than to
have it sitting on your pantry shelf during those vulnerable
first days at home when you might be tempted to feed it to
your baby, thus sabotaging your breastfeeding program.

YOUR MENTAL HEALTH

As the mother of a new baby, you are in one of the most in-
tense periods of your entire life. You're likely to be feeling a
dizzying array of emotions, including excitement, joy, and a
deep sense of inner satisfaction, as well as worry, disappointment, and possibly even depression. You may look at your baby
sometimes, perhaps when you have just been roused from a
deep sleep or when your nipples hurt or when you turn down
an invitation because you can't or don't want to get a baby-
sitter, and think, "Motherhood isn't all it's been cracked up to
be." If you do, you are not alone. Practically every mother alive
has at one time or another had this thought. For no matter
how much you longed to have a child and how much you love
him, he has wrought vast changes in your life.

The birth of a baby marks a major transition point in both
parents' lives, but it's usually much more marked for the
mother, since her life is apt to change more than the new
father's. Even in these "liberated" times, in most homes most
of the responsibility for raising children falls to the mother.
Even if you plan to continue to work outside the home, if
you're typical you'll probably be the parent who finds the
child care and gets your child to the caregiver, who stays home
with a sick child, who keeps track of what needs to be done.
Studies show that married working mothers generally handle
70 to 80 percent of child-care and household responsibilities
in addition to their paying jobs.

The breastfeeding mother is particularly conscious of her

involvement in her baby's care, and her primary responsibility for that care. Even as you love your baby, you may chafe at her complete dependence on you. And as you have these feelings, you're likely to be overwhelmed by guilt because you know that mothers are supposed to love their babies all the time, 24 hours a day, seven days a week.

Many new mothers are guilt-ridden when they realize that they feel no great surge of love when they first see their babies. But maternal love sometimes takes time to develop. In one classic study, only half of a group of 54 new mothers said they had had positive feelings when they first saw their babies (and only 13 percent identified these feelings as love), and about a third reported having had no feelings at all. It took most of the mothers about three weeks to begin to love their babies; by three months the loving tie was usually firmly set.

You may undergo a bout of depression soon after your baby's birth, a syndrome so common it has a name—"postpartum depression" or "the baby blues." This depression usually hits within the first week or two. In fact, it used to be called "milk blues" or "milk fever," because it often seems to accompany the first appearance of milk.

You may find yourself losing your temper or crying at the slightest provocation. You may have problems eating, sleeping, or getting up in the morning. You may lose interest in everything and everybody. To make matters worse, you may worry and feel guilty about the depression itself.

The first thing you need to know is that your reaction is not abnormal. About half of all new mothers have these blues, and second-time mothers are more vulnerable than mothers of first babies. Some experts feel that the changed hormonal balance in the body is to blame, especially in light of the sudden change in hormone levels brought on by the delivery of the baby and placenta. While this sounds sensible, it doesn't explain why only half of newly delivered women experience the depression even though all experience similar hormonal changes. Furthermore, nursing women have higher levels of prolactin, which often is a calming influence, and yet they're just as likely to have the blues.

The answer probably lies in the combination of hormonal changes and changes in your life. If this is your first baby, you have to change the entire rhythm of your days to fit the baby's

Ways to Boost
Your Postpartum Morale

While there's no surefire way to prevent those after-baby blues, many new mothers have found the following measures helpful:

•Take care of yourself. You can't meet your baby's needs if you don't meet your own. (See Chapter 5 for suggestions.)

•Eat well.

•Get plenty of rest. Nap during the day when the baby sleeps to make up for getting up at night.

•If you're used to exercising, gradually get back into a routine. You may not find the time to do all that you did before, but you'll still benefit from doing something. If you haven't exercised before, this would be a good time to start. For one thing, there's evidence that regular exercise releases substances in the body that contribute to feelings of well-being. (See Chapter 5 for suggestions.)

•Forget about housework for the time being.

•Ask for help—from your husband, your relatives, your friends.

needs. Both you and your husband are suddenly catapulted into new feelings of responsibility, and your relationship with him is affected. Even if you already have other children, the arrival of a new baby means new financial responsibilities, new room arrangements, and new routines for the entire family. On top of that, you're probably wondering how you can handle your older children's reactions to the new baby. All this when chronic fatigue is likely to make all the other problems worse. Before you have a baby, it's impossible to know what it will be like, and most women (including adoptive mothers) find that taking care of a newborn is more exhausting and time-consuming than they had ever imagined. As a breastfeeding mother, your sleep is constantly being interrupted and your

●Work out an arrangement so that your husband can spend more time at home and do more in the home for a while.

●Pay for as much help as you can afford. It's a good investment for your comfort and peace of mind.

●Cut back on outside responsibilities.

●Take some time for yourself every day, even if some days it's only 15 minutes to read a magazine.

●Pay attention to your appearance; you'll feel better if you look better. But don't concentrate on your waistline—and, above all, don't try to put on your prepregnancy clothes yet.

●After the first week get dressed every day. At first staying in your robe may help you get your rest, since people won't expect too much of you. After this time, though, it can be dispiriting to find yourself in your bathrobe at 6:00 P.M.

●Join a group for new mothers (such as those sponsored by La Leche League, a childbirth education group, or a local family service agency). You'll find that other mothers have similar problems and feelings and can help with yours.

●You may look at this list and groan, thinking that these suggestions are too much trouble. But many women find that when they exert themselves to take care of themselves, they end up feeling better.

body is working overtime, both to recover from the labor and to feed your baby.

Furthermore, in our society the typical new mother tends to lack self-confidence in her maternal ability. You *know* motherhood must be difficult because there are so many books telling you how to handle your children's psyches, how to raise their IQs—even how to feed them at your breast! And if the professionals disagree about the best theories of child rearing, how are you to have confidence that you know what's best?

These days many women undergo new stresses around motherhood. Having idealized both childbirth and breastfeeding, some women have found that neither experience has lived up to their expectations. They're disappointed with the experience and disappointed in themselves, feeling that they didn't quite measure up. Women who had planned to have a completely unmedicated delivery and then needed some form of anesthetic often forget that the ultimate goal of childbirth is a healthy baby and a healthy mother. Then, in an age when women are urged to have it all, many women learn with a start that combining career with motherhood is much harder than they had expected it to be and feel that there's something wrong with them—rather than the unrealistic expectations abroad in the land these days.

As a breastfeeding mother, your confidence may be further undermined by the fact that you're the exclusive supplier of your baby's food. When a bottle-fed baby cries, or has frequent or sparse bowel movements, or sleeps too little or too much, a mother (and the people around her) will blame the formula or the baby's personal inclinations. In our society, the first reaction is often to blame the breastfeeding. You worry that your baby's not getting enough milk or that your milk isn't good enough or that you're doing something wrong. The unhelpful remarks of other people often feed this anxiety. No wonder your confidence is shaky and your feelings can run away with you!

If you're having major problems with the breastfeeding— if your baby isn't gaining enough or if you have developed a medical condition that makes it very difficult to continue nursing—it's not surprising that you should be upset. Almost always, with the right help you will be able to overcome such difficulties and to move beyond them. If, however, you decide to wean your baby earlier than you had planned to, either for his or your well-being, it's only natural to feel a sense of sadness and disappointment, to mourn for the loss of an experience that was highly meaningful. There is no reason, however, to feel guilty. By nursing for whatever time you did, you gave your baby more than he would have gotten if you had never breastfed him at all.

Be reassured that you are doing the best you can for your baby. Then accept your negative feelings along with your positive ones and realize that you're neither bad nor inadequate for having them. We can't help how we feel about things, even though we can control what we do about our feelings. You'll learn to live with these mixed feelings as you learn to live with mixed feelings about every other aspect of life—your marriage, your work, your schooling. So it is with parenthood. We learn to take the bad with the good—the dirty diapers with the joyous gurgles, the waking up at three in the morning with the bright smile that rewards us as we go to the crib, the burdens of responsibility with the all-embracing love of a child. When you come right down to it, most parents feel that the joys of having and raising children far outweigh the demands they make.

8

You Are a Nursing Couple

No one is ever prepared for the time and energy needed to care for a new baby. No matter how much you've read or how many friends you've spoken to, you get a whole new understanding of what parenthood is all about when you and your own baby are together at home. You probably have more questions now than you did in the hospital, when so much of your life was structured and where a staff of health care providers was at your elbow, ready with answers (even if the answers weren't always that helpful). You're probably more tired now than you ever thought you could be, and you wonder whether you'll ever be back to your old energetic, self-confident self. You will. And you'll get there sooner if you give yourself what we routinely grant our newly elected public officials—a settling-in time for establishing new routines and responsibilities.

Many new mothers impose unrealistically high expectations on themselves. In their eagerness to look upon childbirth as natural (which it is), they forget that recovery from it is natural, too, and that most societies around the world decree a period of rest for the new mother, when she is cared for by others in the community. In their belief in their own strength and competence (which is justified), they deny themselves the means to restore that strength and enhance that competence.

One mother of a one-month-old baby embarrassedly told a visitor, "The baby was up a lot last night and I didn't even get dressed today until three o'clock." She apologized for having a messy house. She fretted because she hadn't resumed her professional contacts. She's a prime example of the modern mother who pushes herself too hard and too fast.

If you can, take the first two or three months after birth as an orientation period. You'll have the time you need to let your body recover from pregnancy and birth and initiate lactation, and to let your psyche get used to the idea of being a mother. Meanwhile, your baby will use this time to get used to the world, to make the big adjustment from having everything done for her in your womb to learning how to do things for herself. The more you can smooth the transition for both of you, the sooner the fun part of mothering and breastfeeding will take over.

Your husband can be enormously helpful at this time. In fact, his involvement can go far toward cementing the two of you as a parenting team, and the three of you as a family. Because of his work commitments, however, and because at this time another woman (especially one who has breastfed) may be able to give a special kind of help, this is the time to call upon one or more people who can serve as your special helper, as described in Chapter 4.

These first few weeks are crucial for the nursing couple. While you don't want to—and you don't have to—shut out the rest of your family and the rest of your life, your primary commitment right now is to your nursing baby and to yourself. You have to feed your baby when he is hungry; you want to rest to help your flow of milk; you have to work at becoming a twosome. Happily, allowing yourself to focus on your baby this way can free you to enjoy him more. By not feeling pressured by other demands, you can give your all to this courtship period. You can consider the worries and the anxieties of these early weeks as akin to the same kinds of tension that often accompany the period of falling in love. Because that is, after all, what the two of you are doing.

DEMAND FEEDING
AT HOME

Probably the first thing you'll want to do after coming home from the hospital or birthing center is to climb into bed and feed your baby. Your milk may just be coming in now if you've been in the hospital for two to five days, or you may have less because of the energy expended in making the trip. If your baby seems fussier and hungrier than she was for the past day or two, this is natural since she has used up some of the body stores she was born with and is now feeling the pangs of hunger. Don't worry: Just rest and nurse frequently, and your milk production will increase.

The concept of "supply and demand" is expressed nowhere more elegantly than in the relationship of the nursing

---

How to Tell
Whether Your Baby Is
Getting Enough Milk

Your baby is probably getting enough milk if:

•In the first month or two she nurses eight to 10 times a day for 10 to 20 minutes on each breast and sleeps for one to three hours between feedings; by the third month she is nursing five to eight times in a 24-hour period and seems contented most of the time.

•He has six or more wet diapers a day with pale yellow urine. Check the wetness of disposable diapers by pinching the bottom of the diaper; if the padding does not spring back to its original shape, the diaper is wet. Also, if it's wet it will feel heavy.

•She has regular bowel movements, either frequent small ones or less frequent large ones.

•He has bright eyes, an alert manner, and good skin tone.

•She is gaining an average of from four to six ounces a week couple. Remember, the more your baby nurses, the more milk you will produce. *The single best thing you can do to ensure successful breastfeeding is to be available to nurse when your baby wants you.*

Still, this is easier said than done. How do you know when your baby wants to nurse, instead of wanting something else? How do you know when your breasts are supplying enough of the milk that your baby is demanding? How can you continue to meet your own needs as an individual? We'll talk about these questions in this chapter and in the next two.

WHEN TO NURSE YOUR BABY

Does demand feeding mean nursing a baby every time he whimpers? It can, but it doesn't have to. As the other half of

---

in the first month and between six to eight ounces a week during the next three months. This gain is apt to vary considerably from week to week. It may range from an ounce or two in one week to a whopping seven or eight ounces the next.

Do not weigh your baby at home. Home-weighing can cause unnecessary worry. Babies' weights fluctuate greatly, and home scales are not accurate. Mothers are sometimes tempted to weigh a baby before and after a feeding to find out how much milk he drank, but controlled experiments with formula-fed babies have found that baby scales tend to underestimate milk intake.

Don't compare your baby's weight gain with other babies. Different babies gain weight at different rates of speed. In the past, formula-fed babies seemed to gain weight faster than the breastfed, but recent research has shown little or no difference between the two groups. Still, there is a considerable range among normal, healthy infants.

Do not test for hunger by offering your baby a bottle after a nursing. Many infants have such a strong urge to suck that they'll often take milk from a bottle even when they are not hungry.

Ways to Build Up Your Milk Production

Following one or more of these suggestions should increase your milk supply within a few days:

• Nurse your baby more frequently for several days, using both breasts at each feeding. This is the *single best way* to enhance your flow of milk.

• Wake your baby sometimes to empty your breasts more often, or pump or express milk between feedings.

• Express or pump milk immediately after each feeding or during feedings if your baby is not suckling well or nurses for only a few minutes at a time.

• Cut back on your schedule. Do less. Relax; rest more. Nap at least once a day, oftener if you can manage it. Maybe you can close your eyes while riding the bus to work or lie down while your older children play quietly nearby. Ask someone else to help with such essentials as marketing, cooking simple meals (or getting take-out food), and doing basic laundry. Take advantage of most people's willingness to help a new mother. You can always reciprocate later on. Ask visitors not to come for a few days unless they'll wait on you, and not expect you to entertain them.

• If possible, take a day or two off from work or from other obligations (by, for example, having someone come in to

the nursing couple, you'll learn how to read your baby's signals. You'll learn to distinguish different kinds of cries—the rhythmic pattern that often means your baby is hungry, the sudden onset of loud crying followed by breath-holding that may indicate pain, or the long, drawn-out wails that communicate frustration. You'll learn when your baby's restless stirring in the crib means that he's about to awaken and when it's just an interlude in sleep. You'll also learn when a smile means that your baby is happily enjoying solitary play, and when one care for your other children) so that you can focus only on feeding the baby.

•Check your diet. Are you eating enough? Some women find that eating more seems to produce more milk. Are you drinking enough fluids?

•Take an extra vitamin B complex. Some nursing mothers have found that one to three teaspoons a day of brewer's yeast helps.

•If the above measures don't work, ask your doctor to prescribe an oxytocin nasal spray to give your let-down reflex (described in Chapter 3) a temporary boost. Sometimes using the spray for a week or two is helpful; longer use, however, is generally ineffective.

•Do *not* offer your baby formula. A few ounces soon turn into a bottle, which soon turns into several bottles, until you find that you're producing even less milk. The only exception is if your baby is sick or so small that his health is endangered, and your doctor (not your friends or relatives) feels that he absolutely needs a supplement. If so, offer it through a nursing supplement like the Lact-Aid™ (described in Chapter 12), or on a spoon.

•Believe in yourself and trust your body. The most effective milk producer of all is nipple stimulation. Tell yourself that millions of other women nurse their babies, and you can, too. The stories you hear of other women who "didn't have enough milk" can almost all be ascribed to lack of information, lack of encouragement, or lack of nipple stimulation.

that appears as you walk into the room means that your company is wanted. This learning is not instinctual; it comes through getting to know your baby and through trial and error. You'll take your cues from your baby and you'll interpret those cues. You'll recognize that your baby's healthy growth depends not only on satisfying his hunger for food and his longing to be held and cuddled, but on his coming to realize that he has the power to influence his world. Responding to signals that your baby sends lets him appreciate this power and build on it in the future. By answering his needs as well as you can when he is small, you'll be setting your child on the road toward becoming secure and independent.

On the other hand, sometimes you'll know what your child needs better than she does. You'll recognize those times when your baby might accept the breast but when she might need some other kind of care even more. And sometimes you'll have to take other considerations, like your own needs and those of other family members, into account. You know that caring for a baby includes but goes beyond offering the breast.

In general, you'll have confidence in your baby's ability to set the pace for nursing and in your ability to keep up with him. You'll nurse the baby whenever he seems to want the breast. He'll want it for the milk, of course. But he'll also appreciate the warmth of your body, the rhythms of your breathing and heartbeat, the comfort of your arms, the feel of your skin on his face.

In the early weeks your baby will probably want to nurse on an average of every two or three hours. He may sometimes sleep for four or five hours between feedings—and at other times want to be fed almost hourly for several feedings. To stimulate your breasts as much as possible and to help your baby go a little longer between feedings, offer both breasts at each nursing.

Babies vary enormously in the feeding schedules they seem to want. Some average 10 to 14 feedings during a 24-hour period for the first month; others are content with eight or even fewer. By one month six to 10 feedings a day constitute a typical range, and by three months some babies cut back to between three and five feedings a day, sleeping through the night, while many others still want to nurse around the clock. Then, just as you seem to see a pattern in your baby's schedule, it's likely to change, possibly because of a spurt in appetite.

Appetite Spurts

Very often babies who have been on fairly regular schedules that everyone seems happy with suddenly begin to clamor for more food. This seems to occur most often at about three weeks, six weeks, three months, and six months of age. Your baby may be undergoing a "growth spurt," a period of rapid growth that makes her especially hungry, or you may be in an "activity spurt," doing so many other things that your body is producing less milk. Whatever the reason, the best way to satisfy your baby's expanded appetite is to nurse more frequently for a few days to increase your milk supply. For other suggestions see the box on page 152 (Ways to Build Up Your Milk Production).

Waking the Baby

Babies are so angelic looking while they're asleep that this is a favorite time for parents to slip into the room, gaze on them with adoration—and express thanks for these precious, peaceful hours. There are some occasions, however, when you may want to gently awaken a sleeping baby:

•**If your baby confuses night with day.** Some babies regularly sleep for five or six hours during the day and then want to be fed almost every hour after you have gone to sleep. You may be able to change the inner "body clock" of a baby by waking him at two- or three-hour intervals during the day; he'll eventually realize that daytime is for nursing and nighttime is for sleep.

•**If your baby is not gaining enough weight.** Some premature babies and others who are unusually docile nurse obligingly when they're up but don't wake up often enough to take in the nourishment they need. In these cases it's sometimes advisable to wake them to increase the number of feedings. For more on the slow-gaining baby, see Chapter 12.

•**If you have scheduling conflicts.** If you expect other children home from nursery school, if you have to go to work, or if something else is going on that would make feeding time hectic and rushed, you may be doing both you and your baby a favor by waking her half an hour or an hour early so that the two of you can enjoy a relaxed quiet nursing.

HOW LONG SHOULD FEEDINGS BE?

We are a clock-watching, number-counting, measuring, and quantifying society. We were this way even before watches with sweep second hands and digital clocks came into common use, and now many of us have to fight the urge to run our lives like train timetables. You can learn from your baby—who does not tell time—and you can use your breastfeeding experience to break minute-hand monarchy and digital despotism.

There is no hard-and-fast rule for establishing the lower or upper limits of a nursing session. Some babies are goal-oriented efficiency experts who milk one breast in five minutes, go on to do the same with the next, and promptly fall asleep. Others nurse and rest, nurse and rest, and want to stay at the breast for an hour or more at a single feeding. Most babies seem to need at least half an hour. Some research indicates that an actively suckling baby will milk each breast in five or six minutes, getting only a trickle the rest of the time. Other research points to multiple let-downs at a single feeding session, with the breasts making milk as long as the baby nurses.

The best way for you to decide when it's time to put your baby down is to watch the baby, not the clock. As we pointed out earlier, you can tell when a baby is actively nursing. Listen for swallowing and look for the working of jaws and temples and the rhythmic sucking in of her cheeks. If you're holding the baby properly and if your nipples are used to the suckling, you can nurse for as long as you and your baby want.

These feeding sessions can be wonderful opportunities to relax, put up your feet, and enjoy being with your baby. Once the nursling is latched on, you might want to watch television or read, or read to a toddler who nestles on one side of you while the baby nurses at the other. If your schedule dictates time limits for some nursings, you can provide a balance by letting others be leisurely.

If your baby never wants to stop nursing, you may want to offer her a pacifier after nursings. It's best not to do this earlier than four to six weeks, however, to prevent nipple confusion. Pacifiers have a long history in baby care; they're good tools

Tips on Relaxing Before and During Feedings

• Telephone a reassuring friend, preferably an experienced nursing mother.

• Eat a healthful snack, such as a small sandwich, piece of fruit, or raw vegetables.

• Drink a glass of water, milk, or juice.

• Lie down for a few minutes ahead of time and nurse lying down.

• Listen to calming music before and during the feeding.

• Read something light and enjoyable.

• Watch a favorite television show.

• Nurse in a quiet room.

• Sit in a comfortable rocker with arms.

• Take an herbal bath or hot shower beforehand.

• Do deep breathing (like the kind you learned in your childbirth class), yoga exercises, visual imagery, or other relaxation techniques before nursing.

• Take an occasional glass of beer or wine, especially before the early evening feeding, which is likely to be the lightest.

• If your nipples are sore, take an occasional aspirin about 30 minutes before you plan to nurse. (See Chapter 12 for suggestions on healing sore nipples.)

for providing extra sucking time for babies who need it, but they should not be used to "plug" a baby's mouth closed every time she opens it or to put her to sleep. By doing that, you may be covering up other needs and creating a hard-to-break habit. There are a great many styles of pacifiers these days, and different babies prefer different shapes. So try one and if your baby rejects it, try other kinds.

IS THE BABY
GETTING ENOUGH MILK?

One of the biggest problems of nursing, in the minds of many women, is that they cannot tell how much milk their babies are drinking. This is actually one of its biggest advantages, since the nursing mother is not tempted to urge her baby to drain the last drop, thus taking more than he wants. If you feed your baby on demand, your supply of milk should keep up with his appetite. If you're well and rested, you're virtually assured of having plenty of milk. Especially if you don't worry too much about it.

After you've been nursing for a while, you'll notice that your breasts are no longer hard and full the way they were at first. This does not mean that you're producing less milk. The glandular changes in the breasts and the increased blood circulation caused their initial fullness. Once milk production is fully established, the breasts become softer and smaller. They remain soft, even while producing copious amounts of milk.

The box on page 150 (How to Tell Whether Your Baby Is Getting Enough Milk) lists some ways to tell whether your baby is getting enough to eat. If you're worried or having trouble with nursing, call a health professional (doctor, nurse, midwife, or lactation consultant), a friend or relative who has breastfeeding experience, or another breastfeeding support person. The person you consult may be able to reassure you over the phone or may want to see you and your baby in person.

IF YOU HAVE
TOO MUCH MILK

Occasionally a woman has such a forceful let-down that her milk spurts clear across the room from the uncovered breast and flows too quickly into the baby's mouth. The baby will gulp noisily, gasp, choke, gag, and sputter during the feeding. He may stop nursing after only a few minutes, only to burst into loud wails of hunger and frustration. A baby forced to drink too quickly from such abundance will swallow air, have uncomfortable air bubbles, hiccup, spit up, and be unable to satisfy sucking needs.

This is easy to correct. If you express the first torrents of milk until it starts to come in a steady drip, your baby will be able to drink more comfortably. Offer just one breast at a feeding. If your other breast becomes uncomfortably full, express or pump the milk and save it either for relief bottles or for contribution to a local milk bank for babies who need more breast milk than their own mothers can supply.

WHEN THE BABY CRIES

Crying is the most powerful way—often the only way—that babies can let the outside world know they need something. It's a vital means of communication and the first way that infants establish any kind of control over their lives.

Research shows that babies whose cries bring relief seem to become more self-confident, seeing that they can affect their own lives. By the end of the first year, babies whose cries have brought tender, soothing care cry less and communicate

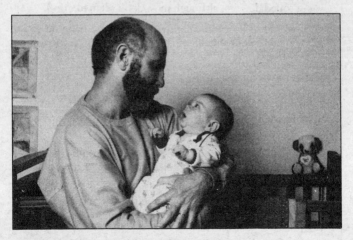

Carrying babies is a time-honored way of soothing them—and the mother isn't the only one who can comfort a crying infant.

Ways to Comfort a Crying Baby

•Pick him up and hold him. Babies probably miss the rhythms of life in the womb, when they felt their mother's heartbeat and breathing all day long. They may be filled with yearnings to be held close and cuddled.

•Sit with the baby in a comfortable rocking chair. A little rocking and cuddling can help you to relax, too.

•If you're nervous and upset, your baby may be responding to your mood. At times like this it's sometimes helpful if someone else can hold the baby for a while. Meanwhile, making extra efforts to put your own cares out of your mind will help you—and may also help your baby. (See Tips on Relaxing Before and During Feedings on page 157.)

•Hold her to your chest vertically with her head over your shoulder and walk her around.

•Change the diaper. Some babies are uncomfortable with wet or soiled diapers, although most don't seem to mind.

•Try switching positions, perhaps moving the baby up so he's lying over your shoulder, his stomach resting on the top of your shoulder.

•Pat or rub her back.

•Burp him. A bubble of air may be causing discomfort.

•Change her position in the crib—to her back, tummy, or side, or with her head where her feet had been.

•Wrap him snugly in a small blanket; some infants feel more secure when firmly swaddled from neck to toes, with arms held close to the sides.

•Make the baby warmer or cooler, either by putting on or taking off clothing or changing the temperature in the room.

•Lay her on her stomach on your chest so she can feel your heartbeat and breathing.

•Give him a massage.

•Give her a warm bath.

•Put him in a baby-pack next to your chest and walk around with him. While you're holding him this way, you can get some of your work done at the same time (like vacuuming, or marketing). Some of these are designed so that you can nurse without taking the baby out of the pack.

•Sing or talk to the baby.

•Provide a continuous or rhythmic sound, like music from the radio, a simulated heartbeat, or "white noise" (a steady background sound) from a whirring fan, vacuum cleaner, or other appliance. You can make a tape recording of one of these sounds.

•Lay him across your knees and move them up and down. This helps many a parent get through dinner.

•Put her in a windup swing seat or cradle. (Some go for as long as 40 minutes.)

•Put springs on the crib legs that turn it into a rocker. At first you can gently rock the baby in it; when he gets bigger he'll be able to do it himself.

•Take the baby out of the house—for a ride in a stroller or car seat—at any hour of the day or night. In bad weather you can walk around in an enclosed mall. The distraction will help you, as well as your baby.

•Lay the baby on top of a folded towel on a washing machine or dryer that's been running for a few minutes. Some babies like the warmth and the motion. You will not, of course, leave his side for even a moment.

•If someone other than the mother is taking care of the baby, it sometimes helps if the caregiver puts on a recently worn item of the mother's clothing (a robe or sweater), so the baby can sense a familiar smell.

•"Dance" with your baby to music from the radio or stereo.

•If the baby seems to have a stomachache (drawing up the
(Continued on the next page)

legs and crying as if in pain), lay him on his back and gently bicycle his legs to help him release gas.

•Hold her in the "colic hold": Stretch her out horizontally on her tummy along your arm, with her head at your elbow and your hand cupped between her slightly dangling legs, holding her by the buttocks or thigh.

•If all else fails, try a pacifier as a last resort. Hold off on doing this until your milk supply is well established, at least four to six weeks after birth, to avoid nipple confusion. Some babies can't work up an interest in pacifiers, but others love them.

•Remember: Having a baby who cries a lot for no discernible reason does not mean that you are an inadequate mother.

more in other ways, while babies of punitive or ignoring caregivers cry more. So don't be afraid of spoiling your baby by going to her when she cries. An infant cannot be spoiled by being picked up and held; the holding itself may be what she's crying for.

When your baby cries two or three hours after the last feeding, you know immediately what to do—bring her to the breast. But suppose she cries an hour after a feeding? Or the minute the feeding ends? What should you do? If this happens during the first few weeks of your baby's life, offer the breast and don't worry about the timing. But if after a month or so, she is regularly waking up and crying more often than every two hours, or if she often cries right after feedings, you'll want to try other ways of comforting her. For suggestions, see the list in the box on the previous pages (Ways to Comfort a Crying Baby).

You cannot, of course, expect to keep your baby from ever crying at all. Frustration and discomfort are a part of life, and part of growing up involves learning how to deal with problems. Babies often fuss in their sleep, find a more comfortable position, and in a few minutes go back to sleeping peacefully. Furthermore, every baby is different. Some babies seem to need to cry lustily for a few minutes before they fall asleep. Unnecessary handling at times like these sometimes overstimulates these babies, interferes with their falling asleep, and makes them cry even more from fatigue. Furthermore, constant parental management can get in the way of babies' solving their own problems.

Babies do cry less when they're carried around, however. Both child care professionals and casual observers have noticed that babies in cultures where their mothers carry them around most of the day seem to cry less than babies in western societies. In industrialized societies, babies generally increase their crying until six weeks of age, then gradually cry less up to four months of age, crying mostly in the evenings. Recently, a team of Canadian researchers conducted an experiment that could revolutionize baby care in the western world. They asked some mothers to carry their babies in their arms or in a baby carrier for at least three hours a day, and they asked others to place a mobile and an abstract picture of a face where the babies could see them from their cribs. The results: the babies who were carried cried less than the ones who were not carried this often.

If your baby seems to be crying "all the time," or for long, unhappy periods at all different times of the day, and nothing that you can do will comfort her, call your doctor. The crying may stem from a problem serious enough to merit medical attention. Most likely, you'll be reassured that your baby is healthy, and you may receive some suggestions for making her—and the rest of the family—more content.

THE COLICKY BABY

Some babies become fussy practically every day in the late afternoon or early evening, and nothing you do can quiet them. Often it's hard to know why this happens—the baby may get tired late in the day or may be responding to the fatigue of other family members or to late-day tension in the household. Most babies magically outgrow this daily crankiness sometime between six weeks and three months of age. Meanwhile, even when they don't seem to respond to your efforts to cheer them up, it's worth continuing to try, since they're getting a sense that the people around them care about how they feel and are there for them.

Often this kind of regular crying stems from physical discomfort, possibly due to an immature gastrointestinal tract. You can see this in the baby who draws up his legs and screams as if in severe pain. It's paradoxical that the typical colicky baby is an eager nurser who's gaining well, who feeds quickly, and who spits up a little bit of milk after every feeding. It's also noteworthy that colic does not seem to be related to personality, since many babies who cry a lot in early infancy turn out to have cheerful, sunny dispositions later on.

If your baby seems to suffer the stomach upset typical of colic, the problem may lie in how the baby eats or in what you eat. Does she gulp furiously, swallowing air? Does your milk come too quickly? If so, see page 158 (If You Have Too Much Milk). Also, take a look at your diet. Recent research has pointed to substances that a nursing mother eats, especially cow's milk, as a cause of colic. When mothers eliminate cow's milk products from their own diets, their babies' symptoms sometimes go away. Other foods in the mother's diet that sometimes seem to cause trouble are eggs, citrus fruits, wheat products, and chocolate. None of these foods is indispensable. As the charts in Chapter 5 show, many different foods are good sources for essential nutrients.

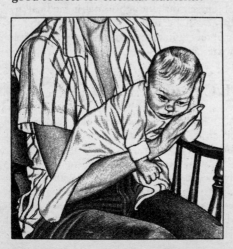

Uncomfortable babies are often soothed by this "colic hold."

Other cases of colic don't seem to be linked to anything the mother eats or anything she does. In many cases the parents are relaxed (at least until the crying jags begin) and experienced (since this isn't their first baby). Yet still their babies cry. So do what you can, don't blame yourself, and look forward to that happy day when the colic will be just a notation in your child's baby book.

You won't be a bad mother if you occasionally turn the baby over to another loving caregiver for a little while so that you can get some relief. This is one great benefit of having other hands to rock the cradle. As the late Margaret Mead said, as an advocate of a system by which several people take turns caring for a baby, "The worst thing is just having the mother boxed up with the baby 24 hours a day, which nobody ever meant to have happen in the whole history of the human race."

NIGHT FEEDINGS

It's the middle of the night, and everyone, including the family dog, is sleeping peacefully. Everyone, that is, except your new baby, whose lusty bawling pierces your sleep. You wonder when that happy day will come when you can once again know a night of uninterrupted sleep. This is hard to say.

The age at which babies give up night feedings seems to be an individual characteristic unrelated to size at birth, weight gain afterwards, the amount of food eaten in a day; or whether this food comes from breast, bottle, or jar. Babies seem to be born with differing needs for sleeping and eating. While the average newborn sleeps about 16 hours a day, one healthy baby may sleep only 11 hours, while another sleeps 21. After three months babies become more wakeful in late afternoon and early evening, and by six months more than half their sleep takes place at night.

An occasional baby gives up middle-of-the-night feedings as early as six weeks; many give it up at about three months; and some need it for several months longer. In the early weeks you need that night feeding as much as your baby does, so that your breasts will continue to be well stimulated and will not become engorged and uncomfortable by morning.

Gradually your baby will go longer between night feedings until one morning you'll wake up, breasts full, wondering what's the matter. Nothing is wrong; your baby has just slept through the night for the first time.

Night feedings are a little easier if you don't bother changing the baby's diapers unless he's absolutely drenched or seems uncomfortable. If a diaper change is necessary, the father can do this. Meanwhile, you'll be getting your rest.

Different families handle sleeping arrangements and nighttime feedings in different ways. The following are the most common:

•For the first month or so, when the baby is waking up several times a night, he sleeps in a crib or cradle next to the mother's bed. As soon as she hears him begin to cry, she reaches over, brings him into bed with her, nurses him, and puts him back to bed. After about a month the baby sleeps in a separate room.

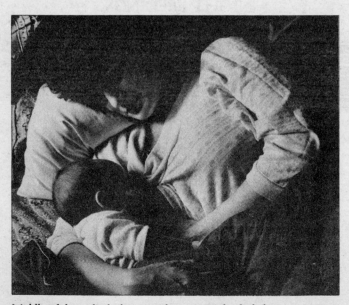

Middle-of-the-night feedings can be cozy (and a little less tiring) when mother takes baby into bed with her.

•The baby sleeps in her own room right from the start. If the parents are afraid they won't hear her cry, they rig an intercom system between their room and the baby's. As soon as she starts to cry, the father gets out of bed and brings the baby to the mother. After the baby has been nursed, the father takes her back to her own bed.

•The baby sleeps in the same bed with the parents. While this practice used to be frowned upon as a safety hazard for fear that mothers or fathers would roll over on their babies, this fear seems to have been ill-founded, and many families find that this enables mothers to respond to their babies most comfortably during the night.

Whichever way you decide to arrange your family life is up to you. So far there's no evidence to prove that any one way is better. Babies grow up happy and healthy under all of the above and a variety of other sleeping arrangements as well. Basically, your choice will depend on your own views of parenting and marriage, and on your own personal preference.

The Joys of Nighttime Feedings

It's hard for an exhausted new mother to think of night feedings as being anything but a burdensome sleep-robber to be ended as soon as possible. Yet many women have found that they welcome and enjoy them more than they ever thought they would—especially if they're able to nap during the day.

Women who like night feedings usually cite emotional reasons. They talk about the warm feeling of nursing in bed, surrounded by the people they love. They talk about the special feeling of being the only two people awake in the house. They talk about the serenity of being alone with their babies. They talk about the slightly illicit feeling of slipping out of bed in the middle of the night and sitting with the baby and a snack in front of a late TV show. "I feel like I'm on a date at a drive-in movie," one mother said. Other mothers who long for these nighttime feedings to end often find with some surprise that years later they look back upon them with nostalgia.

Encouraging a Baby to Give Up Nighttime Nursing

If you don't really mind getting up at night, there's no age by which the baby has to sleep through, so you can just wait until he gives up night feedings himself—and try to catch up on your own sleep by scheduling a nap during the day. But if the baby is a good size and is nursing often and well during the day (if he's at least eight weeks old, so that your milk supply is well established), and if getting up with him leaves you exhausted and irritable, you may be able to encourage him to sleep for longer stretches at night. Sometimes one of the following will work:

• Try nursing later at night, maybe at midnight, to see whether this will hold the baby till morning.

• Let the baby fuss (not scream) for 15 to 20 minutes when he wakes up during the night; if he's not too hungry, he may go back to sleep.

• Let your husband go in to comfort the baby, maybe by rubbing her back or rocking her in her crib. From a very early age, your baby associates your looks and your smell with feeding; if you go in, she'll expect to nurse. This is why the father or someone else may be more successful in getting her back to sleep.

• If your baby is on a "night shift," sleeping during the day and up a lot at night, reorient him by waking him up and nursing him every two or three hours during the day, and keeping him awake by taking him out, bathing him, playing with him or sitting him in an infant seat where he can see interesting things and people.

• While some parents feed their babies solid foods in the belief that this will help them go longer between nursings at night, there's no evidence that this does any good. So you should continue giving your baby breast milk alone for four to six months. (Suggestions for starting solids are given in Chapter 14.)

• Offer a pacifier.

DIAPERS, REVISITED

Remember that your baby's bowel movements and habits are quite different from those of a bottle-fed baby. A grandmother or friend used to bottle-fed babies may look at your baby's stools, become worried about his health, and alarm you. So put their minds and your own at ease.

Your baby may move his bowels quite frequently, possibly after every feeding. Or he may move them only once a day, or once every three or four days. Or he may start out one way and change his patterns of elimination. (Breastfed babies tend to excrete less waste than formula-fed infants, because human milk is digested so completely.)

The movements of a breastfed baby are usually soft, seedy, and yellowish. They've been described as being like soft scrambled eggs with a little water around them or like a mixture of cottage cheese and mustard. Sometimes there's only a stain on the diaper; this is not diarrhea. Sometimes your baby strains a bit; this is not constipation. All these patterns are normal and healthy.

Your baby's stools may become looser in response to something you have eaten—large quantities of fruit juice, for example, or certain foods in the cabbage family. Try to discover the offending food and avoid it. Do not take any strong laxative, because this can give your baby diarrhea.

While constipation is rare among breastfed babies, it occasionally appears. If your baby goes a week without moving her bowels or if she seems to be in pain when she does, there are several things you can do. One is to drink six ounces of prune juice or eight ounces of apple juice once or twice a day. Another is to eliminate cow's milk from your diet and see what happens. If neither of these steps helps, call your doctor.

To prevent infection in either you or your baby, wash your hands after diapering and before nursing him.

YOUR SOCIAL LIFE

While you're getting started at breastfeeding, you'll probably find that the only social life you're interested in for a while revolves around making friends with your baby and integrating the newcomer into the family. This is just as well since you need your rest and the freedom from outside pressures. Still, the time will come when you want to see friends and go places. There's no reason why you can't.

Going Out With the Baby

Once your baby is three or four weeks old, you can get out for an occasional visit with friends or a trip to a nearby restaurant—and you can take the baby with you. Babies this young are usually very agreeable to going out and bedding down for a while in carriage, carrier, or car-bed. Should your nursling want to be fed, you're right there. The only danger about this is that it seems so easy that you may tend to overdo it. If you find that you're going out so often and staying out so late that you or your baby is getting tired and irritable, cut back.

Going Out Without the Baby

By the time your milk supply is well established and your baby has developed a regular enough schedule so that you can sometimes predict when she'll want to be fed (perhaps between six weeks and three months), you may want to go out from time to time without the baby. You may miss an occasional afternoon or evening feeding, but it's best to miss as few as possible, preferably no more than one or two a week if you don't have to. You don't want your baby to develop a preference for the bottle. If you do plan to be away from your baby sometimes, offer an occasional bottle from the age of six weeks on; otherwise your baby may refuse to take one later on. (Some of the suggestions offered working mothers in Chapter 9 may be applicable.)

If possible, express or pump your milk when you're away. When you feel a let-down or at the time you would ordinarily nurse, find a private spot where you can express. You'll feel more comfortable, you'll be less likely to leak, and the breasts will get the regular stimulation they need to keep producing milk.

When you leave a relief bottle (which you should not do, if possible, before your baby is six weeks old), you can leave your own breast milk which you have previously expressed and refrigerated or frozen. Or you can leave a bottle of ready-to-feed formula. Your baby should not be drinking plain homogenized cow's milk until at least six months of age, and preferably one year. (For information on expressing, storing, and freezing breast milk, see the Appendix.)

Nursing in Public

Many women nurse their babies wherever they happen to be—but with such deftness that no one else is aware of what they're doing. Still, if you feel shy about nursing in front of other people, you don't have to. When feeding time comes, excuse yourself, go into another room, and feed the baby. Or start the baby nursing in another room and then rejoin the group. (Usu-

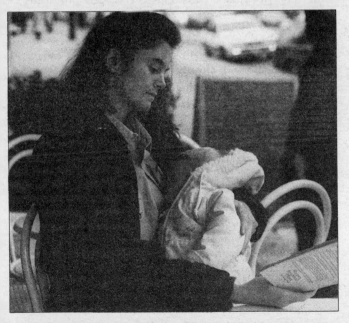

More American women are nursing wherever their daily lives take them, with the confidence that they are doing the best they can for their babies.

ally the time your breast is most exposed is at the start of a feeding. Once the baby has latched on, it's easier to keep your breast covered.) Most people will respect your privacy. In a public place where you can't be alone, you can usually find a quiet nook where you'll be relatively unobserved. Or an adult with you may be able to shield you from public view.

However, if you feel comfortable about breastfeeding in front of others, there's no reason why you shouldn't. You need not feel apologetic or bashful about nurturing your baby the way mothers have done from the dawn of history. While denying maternal sexuality, our society's erotic interest in the female breast has generated a taboo against showing it in public, thus keeping many women from nursing. The sight of a mother suckling her infant—sanctified in paintings of the Madonna and Child and accepted on the streets of less "civilized" countries around the world—is considered indecent in much of the western world.

Columnist Ann Landers tells women not to nurse their babies in the presence of guests in their own homes. Nursing mothers have been evicted from restaurants, hotels, and swimming pool enclosures. But why should a woman have to sequester herself from normal life and from other adults because she wants to do the best thing for her baby?

More and more women are refusing to accept this taboo. They're nursing their babies in meetings, at parties, at concerts and ballgames, on beaches, on airplanes, and in church and synagogue. More contemporary observers are becoming familiar with a sight that was once commonplace in Western society and is once again regaining its proper place as an acceptable practice. As women themselves accept the naturalness and the respectability of breastfeeding, societal acceptance of public nursing will keep apace.

Furthermore, good wardrobe planning can help you breastfeed so discreetly that no one has to even see your breasts. You can cover more of you by unbuttoning your blouse from the bottom up rather than from the top down. Knit pullovers can be easily pulled up so that the baby's body will cover your midriff and the pullover will cover your breast. Ponchos, loose-fitting cardigan sweaters and jackets, scarves, and shawls are all good coverups. You may want to practice nursing at home with different kinds of clothes until you feel comfortable about doing it in public. (Also see Clothes for the Nursing Mother in Chapter 5.)

YOUR OLDER CHILDREN

If you have other children, you may wonder about their reactions to your nursing the new baby. You may be afraid that your feeding the baby in such an intimate way will make them jealous. Actually, your older children, especially the one closest in age to the new one, will have ambivalent feelings toward the new baby, no matter how you feed. This doesn't seem any worse when the baby is nursed.

You can expect your older ones to be on your lap or by your side as the baby is nursing. (We're not talking here about toddlers whom you nursed after you became pregnant again and are still "tandem" nursing, which we'll say more about in Chapter 13, but about those who were never nursed or were weaned some time back.) Accept this and make feeding times family times. One advantage of breastfeeding is that you have a free arm with which to draw your toddler close to you or to turn the pages of her favorite book. While the infant has your breast, your older child has your attention on his level. Show your other children in many ways that the new baby has not displaced them in your affection, but don't let them feel that they have the right to deprive the infant of the right to be nursed.

Occasionally toddlers ask whether they can nurse, too. If you let your child try, he'll probably laugh and forget about it or may even put his mouth to the breast and then not know what to do about it. The suckling movements that come so naturally to a newborn seem to be easily forgotten. Many babies forget how to do it as soon as a month after they have been weaned. If your toddler is different, though, and does want to go back to nursing, you can point out to him that this is something that only little babies do—and you can follow this by giving him a treat that is only for "*big* boys" (or "girls").

If you breastfed your older children, you can tell them that you fed them this way when they were babies and that now it's the new baby's turn. If you did not breastfeed them, there's no need to volunteer this information, but if they're old enough and curious enough to ask you about it, be truthful. Explain that when they were little you didn't know how good breastfeeding was for the baby and for the mother. Now that you do know, you want to be as good a mother as you can to the new baby, just as you want to be a good mother to all your children. Most youngsters accept a simple explanation like this, and are happy to hear that even adults keep learning new things.

As a breastfeeding mother you have a lovely opportunity to provide some elementary sex education in an easy, natural way. The child who sees his little brother or sister at the breast learns some of the biological differences between men and women, and gains a sense of the function and beauty of the human body. Your little daughter may be especially inspired by the thought that she will be able to care for her babies in this special way when she grows up.

Your older children can probably offer more help to you than you realize. Take advantage of their interest in being eager baby-amusers, willing fetch-and-carriers, and pleasant companions to you as they help you fold the laundry, set the table, or push the baby carriage. Some of the happiest family times occur in such everyday activities.

WHAT IS YOUR BABY LIKE?

All new babies have certain characteristics in common. They all have facial configurations particularly suited for nursing—the receding chin and flat nose that let them get their faces in the right position at the breast and the well-developed cheek muscles they need for suckling. They all cry when they want something, eat often, and need to be taken care of. They're all tiny, dependent, defenseless, and appealing.

However, we now know scientifically what parents have always known—that each baby comes into this world with a unique personality. Studies that have followed children from birth into adulthood have found that individuals differ enormously right from the beginning in such characteristics as activity level; regularity in biological function (hunger, sleep, and elimination); adaptability to change; acceptance of new situations; sensitivity to noise, light, and other sensory stimulation; mood (cheerfulness or crankiness); distractibility; intensity of feelings and responses; and persistence.

As parents, we don't have the power to turn out children who behave in certain ways. Furthermore, children's temperaments influence the way we respond to them. A cheerful baby is treated differently from a fussy one, an active one from a docile one, and a predictable one from one with very irregular patterns.

Since you'll respond to your baby's personality, it's helpful to think about his temperament and to accept his uniqueness as an individual. You may recognize your child immediately in the following profiles, or decide he's a combination of several, or realize that his personality is different from anything described here. Whichever way your baby is, the important thing for you to do is to accept and love him for the way he is, not for the way you would like him to be.

The Alarm Clock. She has an inner clock that wakes her regularly, about every three hours at first. She sleeps about the same time every day, tends to move her bowels at the same time every day, and in general has predictable patterns. She's easy to live with, easy to take care of.

The Nonconformist. This is the baby who tries parents' souls. He sleeps for two hours one morning, for 15 minutes the next, and not at all the third. He's ravenously hungry Monday morning and totally uninterested on Tuesday. He offers few clues to his wants. If left to set his own demand feeding schedule, he innocently runs his mother ragged. This child benefits from parental guidance in helping to regularize his living patterns.

The Good Eater. She comes to the breast with a good appetite and an inborn knowledge of technique. She eats well, sucking so vigorously that she develops blisters on the middle of both upper and lower lips. These don't bother the baby; the skin falls off, another blister forms, and the cycle repeats itself till the baby's lips become hardened to her energetic nursing.

The Waiter. He doesn't become interested in nursing until about the fourth or fifth day. He may be sleepy from childbirth medication, or he may not feel like exerting himself until his mother's milk comes in.

The Dawdler. She's a slow eater who nurses for a few minutes, then rests awhile. Other times she mouths the nipple, tastes the milk, and then sets to work. She takes the milk in her own good time and cannot be hurried.

The Dozer. He likes to sleep, especially at mealtimes. You may be able to rouse him by dabbing him on the forehead with a sponge dampened with cool water, expressing a little milk into his mouth, taking off some of his clothing, leaning him forward on your lap, walking your fingers up his spine, or massaging his legs and arms. Playing with him before a feeding may encourage him to stay awake and changing diapers after the first breast may wake him up enough to take the second.

The Overeager Beaver. She becomes so excited at feeding time that she moves her head quickly from side to side, grasps the breast, then loses it and ends up screaming in frustration. Handle her gently, speak to her softly, keep putting her back on the breast. Try to nurse her before she gets frantically hungry, even if you have to wake her sometimes to do it. Eventually she gets the idea and settles in.

The Biter. He comes down hard on your breast, chewing it as if he had been born with a mouthful of teeth. When he starts chewing, withdraw your breast; break the suction with your finger. Even an infant can learn not to bite the breast that feeds him. A baby who is actively nursing cannot bite.

If your baby starts to bite when he's teething, take your breast away and say "No!" firmly every time he tries to bite. Don't make a game of it. Another trick that sometimes works is to say the baby's name quietly while drawing him close to you; this distracts him and gets him back to nursing. Give him special teething toys and foods. If he keeps biting, keep your finger close to his mouth and watch him carefully; as soon as he stops nursing actively or looks playful, remove your breast. He'll get the idea.

The Spitter. Fat and healthy, she spits up milk after practically every feeding. She may continue this until she's almost a year old and you're convinced that you, the baby, and the apartment will always smell cheesy. (The smell is a lot milder while she's on breast milk alone.) Try propping her at a 30-degree angle for a while after nursing before you try to burp her. This helps the milk settle in the stomach and discourages it from coming up with the air bubble.

The Lopsided Nurser. He develops a preference for one of your breasts. He's not lopsided, but you soon get that way. If one breast is producing more milk than the other, offer the less full one first at every feeding: The baby will drain it better and encourage it to produce more; when it does, you can go back to alternating. Also try to switch nursing positions· Hold the baby more vertically or in the football hold, or nurse lying down. If you can't influence him to give both breasts equal treatment, forget about it and pad your bra on the smaller side when you go out. When you stop nursing you'll regain your symmetry.

The Playboy/Playgirl. Practically every baby falls into this category at some time—usually at about four or five months. By this time they're more aware of the world around them and eager to show how much they love you. He'll suddenly pull away in the middle of a feeding to flash you a bright toothless smile. Or she'll turn her head in response to a voice or footstep. He'll stroke your breast or face with his dimpled little hand. She'll play with the buttons on your blouse. This is such a beautiful way to cement a loving relationship that you should make every effort to relax and enjoy these longer, more playful feedings. If you occasionally want the feeding to go more quickly, nurse in a dark, quiet room free from distractions.

It takes a couple of months for you and your baby to become attuned to each other. The first few weeks you're both busy learning how to nurse and the next few, you're perfecting the art. During this time you come to know what to expect of your life together. You learn that there are days when everything goes smoothly—and days when nothing does. You learn that there are days when your baby is cranky and days when you're cranky. You know that you can cope with all these ups and downs because that's what life is all about. By the time these first couple of months have passed, the trial-and-error period is over. You don't have long lists of questions about breastfeeding. You know what to do—and you go about doing it. You and your baby are a nursing couple.

How long will you remain a nursing couple? This is up to you and your baby, a matter of personal preference, life-style, philosophy, and personality. In Chapter 14 we'll talk about some of the choices you can make in deciding when to wean your baby. Till then we'll explore other facets of the life of the nursing couple.

9

The Working
Nursing Mother

Over the past couple of decades we have seen two major changes in women's lives. The year 1969 marked a turning point in the history of American women, as for the first time more mothers of school-age children were holding down jobs than were working as full-time homemakers. Since then the proportion of mothers in the workplace has continued a steady rise, with the biggest increase in recent years among mothers of children under the age of three. More than 40 percent of today's working mothers have children under one year of age.

The year 1971 marked a different kind of turning point, as the year marking the lowest breastfeeding rates in this country in history. Since then the proportion of women choosing to nurse their babies has also risen steadily. As these two trends have come together, then, we have an increasing number of women who are working outside the home and are also nursing their babies.

Yes, it can be done, many women are doing it, and what's more, many women are enjoying combining these two activities. Many working mothers express a special appreciation of the joys of breastfeeding. Away from their babies for much of the day, they savor the special warmth and intimacy of the nursing relationship when they are home. They find that the intensity of the nursing experience helps to make up for the hours they are away from their families. Furthermore, many working mothers find that the ability to sit and nurse actually has a calming, relaxing effect on them, while reminding the baby who the real mother is!

Not that it's easy. Anyone who combines working for pay and caring for a family is bound to experience one conflict after another, growing out of limited reserves of time and energy. Adding breastfeeding to the daily schedule imposes still another layer of activities and concerns. Yet more and more women are so convinced of the value of breastfeeding and are so committed to their work (for reasons of personal fulfillment, economic necessity, or both) that they are determined to carry out both activities. A few years back women were saying, "I'm going back to work. Can you help me wean my baby?" Now they say, "I'm going back to work. Can you help me keep on nursing?"

How do so many women manage to combine these areas of their lives so well? They line up the support they need—and they organize their lives for success.

FINDING SUPPORT

This is one time in your life when you need as much help as you can get. Your time to assist others will come, but for now you have to reach out for the aid that others can give you. Help is where you find it.

If your husband takes over some of the household chores, cares for your baby in many important ways, and provides that all-important dollop of moral support that lets you know you're doing a good job, you're lucky. (Of course this is only fair. If you're helping to win the bread, he should be helping to make the home.) If your husband provides verbal support for your efforts but not much more, you may be able to enlist his cooperation by letting him know how important his help is to your success at breastfeeding. (Ask him, for example, to read Chapter 11 in this book.) If he still does not do as much as you would like him to, you may need to look for help elsewhere.

You may be able to call upon your baby-sitter for help above and beyond the work she was hired for. Or you may be able to go to family members. (One mother told us, for example, of a time when she had to visit her husband in the hospital. She met her brother after work, he took her expressed milk, picked up the baby at the sitter, and gave the baby the bottle.) Don't forget friends, neighbors, coworkers, employers, or local support groups like La Leche League, Childbirth Education Association, or ASPO/Lamaze. It's especially important for single mothers to find people to help them through this gratifying, though demanding, period of their lives.

If your income permits extras or if anyone wants to give you a generous baby gift, there's no better use for money at this time than hiring someone to do the cleaning, the cooking, the laundry, and so forth, an investment that can pay off in your physical and psychological comfort, and ultimately in the entire family's well-being.

The special helper we talked about in Chapter 4 can be a life-saver for the working mother. She (or he) can step in at times of emergency and lighten your load in many ways on a day-to-day basis. If you don't have someone in your life to serve this function, you may need to call upon some of the problem-solving abilities that serve you so well on the job to locate one or more people to share that all-important task.

PLANNING AHEAD: WHILE YOU'RE PREGNANT AND STILL ON THE JOB

The time to arrange for your maternity leave and to enlist your employer as your ally is during your pregnancy. Actually, the first step in your campaign should have come *before* your pregnancy—when you performed your work so well and made yourself so valuable to your employers that they are eager to do whatever is necessary to bring you back and keep you happy. Highly valued employees can often obtain all sorts of concessions that company policy ordinarily prohibits, such as longer maternity leaves, temporary part-time schedules, and the opportunity to do some of your work at home. If your position with your company is strong, ask for whatever you want. You may be pleasantly surprised at what you can get.

A Model Program for Working Breastfeeding Mothers

In view of the many health advantages that breastfeeding confers on both mothers and babies, it's highly appropriate that a hospital should have pioneered in offering a special program to affirm its commitment to encourage breastfeeding among its employees. Yet the kind of program instituted in 1980 by the Hunterdon Medical Center in Flemington, New Jersey,[1] could be undertaken by many organizations that employ sizable numbers of women. It's the kind of program that workers could urge their employers to adopt.

Besides benefiting breastfeeding families, the program serves employers, too. Women who have used it have said that it made their return to work physically easier, some said they would not have come back to work if the pump had not been available, some came back earlier than they had planned to, and others were able to work longer hours.

The program includes the following features:

• A three-month maternity leave policy, with readily granted extensions.

• An electric breast pump kept in the office of the employee health service, accessible on any work shift. The health service nurse informs women who take maternity leave about the pump and shows those who are interested in using it when they come back to work where it is and how it works. She also teaches them techniques for storing and using their breast milk at home.

[1]Katcher, A. L. and Lanese, M. G. (1985). "Breast-Feeding by Employed Mothers: A Reasonable Accommodation in the Work Place," Pediatrics, 75 (4): 644–647.

Your Maternity Leave

As a responsible employee, you will need to tell your employer about your pregnancy before you show up in a maternity dress and before you tell your coworkers. Fairly early in your preg-

•A refrigerator kept in the health service office to store milk, and a sink and a water source for rinsing equipment.

•A nurse especially knowledgeable about breastfeeding who is available for advice. (This role could also be assumed by a lactation consultant or an experienced nursing mother.)

Administrators of this program recommend that any employer who wants to institute a similar one include the following features:

•A policy, agreed upon by department heads, senior administrators, and employees, that recognizes women's responsibilities to both job and family.

•A person knowledgeable about lactation designated to help mothers during their leaves and after they return to work.

•A place set aside for breast milk expression that is easily accessible and yet not disruptive of daily work schedules. It should provide privacy, comfort, and good ventilation.

A society like ours, which proclaims its commitment to families, should express that commitment by providing services that help parents give their children the best care possible. In this regard we lag far behind some other countries. In Sweden, for example, new mothers receive 90 percent of their salary for nine months and may ask for nine months more of unpaid leave, with their job guaranteed. Of more than 100 countries surveyed in 1975, 75 percent had laws requiring nursing breaks and child care in or near the mother's workplace. Our government could do much more to encourage employers to institute family-oriented policies. Providing tax incentives to businesses that institute programs like this one, that provide day care assistance, and that help families in other ways is one goal we should work for.

nancy you'll want to ask for an appointment with your supervisor to discuss your plans and your future with the company. Tell her how long you expect to continue working and how much maternity leave you plan to take.

The absolute minimum for your maternity leave should be four weeks, and the more you can negotiate for (either paid or unpaid), the easier it will be for you. A good goal to shoot for is four to six months. With this amount of time, you'll be well rested by the time you go back to work, your milk supply will be well established, and your baby is more apt to be sleeping through the night and on a fairly predictable schedule.

One study of 567 working breastfeeding mothers, whose occupations covered a wide range (including mill and factory workers, police officers, postal carriers, secretaries, preschool through college-level teachers, business executives, attorneys, and physicians), found that the typical time of return to work was 10 weeks after birth, and that three-fourths of these women were back on the job before their babies were 13 weeks old. Those who returned before the baby's fourth month were likely to wean earlier than those who stayed home longer.[2]

Furthermore, those mothers who didn't go back to work until their babies were four months old were less likely to feel that their employment affected their breastfeeding negatively. Still, 40 percent of the "early" returners continued to nurse past their babies' first birthday. So even if you have to go back to work earlier than you would like, you can still have a successful breastfeeding experience.

Your Breastfeeding Plans

It's not necessary to discuss your breastfeeding plans when you first speak to your employer. After all, that time is a long time away. Besides, your employer may not be interested in discussing them with you. In fact, depending on the atmosphere at your workplace, you may decide never to discuss your nursing with anyone there, but instead to privately work out your own arrangements. Many women have found, however, that talking with their employers ahead of time was helpful in enlisting

---

[2]This study, by Kathleen G. Auerbach, Ph.D. and Elizabeth Guss, specified only one cut-off point to differentiate early and late weaning—the first birthday. Therefore we can assume that many of these "early-weaning" mothers nursed as long as six or nine months, ages that in our society are not generally considered early weaning. (See Chapter 14 for a discussion of different ages for weaning.)

support and in providing reassurance that the job was still important to them.

Good times to talk about these plans are just before you go on leave or just before you plan to return. If you do raise the issue of your nursing, you will want to make the following points:

•Breastfeeding is not totally time-consuming. Most likely you know other working women who have found it compatible with their work schedules, and you are organizing your life so you can handle it, too. At this time you can talk about how you plan to express your milk (whether you'll use your coffee and lunch breaks for this and where you might go for privacy and comfort) and how you plan to make up any extra time you might need (by coming in early, staying late, or taking lunch at your desk.)

•Breastfeeding mothers need not be restricted. With good organization, nursing women can be away from their babies if necessary for the complete work day (and sometimes even longer, although this is certainly a situation you don't want to encourage.)

•In terms of your lifetime career, the period of time you'll be breastfeeding is really very short. You have shown your commitment to your work up until now, and this will continue long after this important temporary interlude.

•Since breastfed babies are usually healthier than bottle-fed babies, you're likely to lose less time from work because of childhood illnesses than you might otherwise. This benefits the employer.

•If your employer's work force includes a large number of young women, you might want to suggest that management consider adopting a program such as the one described in the box on page 182 (A Model Program for Working Breastfeeding Mothers). Such a program is inexpensive and easy to install. Yet it can go far toward attracting new workers, shortening the maternity leaves of the ones who are already there, and increasing productivity by increasing morale.

PLANNING AHEAD: WHILE YOU'RE ON YOUR MATERNITY LEAVE

While most of your efforts during this brief time will probably involve getting used to caring for a new baby, establishing the breastfeeding relationship, and resting after the labor of childbirth, you will want to use these weeks at home to handle some important steps.

Finding Child Care

The first is finding good child care—if you didn't already make your arrangements during your pregnancy.[3] For some specific suggestions on establishing a caregiving relationship that supports your nursing relationship, see the box on page 187 (Finding Child Care That Will Support Your Plans to Breastfeed).

Introducing the Bottle

Since the key to your success in combining working and breastfeeding will probably lie in your baby's having one or more bottle-feedings while you're at work, it's vital that you take special pains to help him like the bottle, even if he doesn't love it. (He'll be saving his love for you.)

By and large, the earlier a baby is given a bottle, the more readily she will take it. Babies confronted with their first bottle at several months of age often refuse it absolutely and will sooner go hungry rather than drink from this strange, unwelcome container so different from their mother's warm breast. A baby five months or older can get supplemental milk from a cup. Yet there is a danger in introducing the bottle *too* early. While some babies have no trouble taking a daily bottle along with the breast feedings right from birth, other babies who are

---

[3]Because this issue has so many ramifications and is so important, we can't go into it in depth here. In these pages we'll talk about child care only as it relates to your breastfeeding plans. For a detailed description of different kinds of care and ways of evaluating them, see: *The Working Parents Survival Guide* by Sally Wendkos Olds (1986). New York: Bantam.

Finding Child Care That Will Support Your Plans to Breastfeed

As a working mother, the most important person in your life after your husband and child is likely to be the person who takes care of that child. As a mother who wants the best possible care for her child, you need to find a caregiver who is both caring and capable. You also need to find someone who will support your breastfeeding plans, not sabotage them.

When you interview a potential caregiver, be sure to let her know that you plan to breastfeed your baby. Be alert to her responses: Does she seem to think this is a wonderful idea or a terrible one? Does she seem to feel that her domain is being invaded? Does she feel that it's a mistake for a working mother to nurse? If you get any clues to such feelings, you'll know that this person is not for you.

If she does seem responsive, however, you need to ask some more questions and to give her some information. Tell her the kind of schedule you have in mind, how many bottles a day you want her to give your baby, how to store the milk, and how to thaw it if you'll be providing frozen milk. Ask whether she has ever taken care of a breastfed baby. If not, you need to tell her about the differences in feeding schedules (breastfed babies eat more frequently), in bowel movements (looser and either more or less frequent, depending on your own baby's pattern) and in ways of soothing the baby (for example, avoiding bottles of water and pacifiers). You may want to give or lend her a copy of this book, marking the pages she's most likely to refer to. Or you can write out the information she needs and put it in a convenient place.

If this person will be coming to your home, ask her to come some time before you go back to work so she can get to know the baby, as well as you and your routines. If you will be taking the baby to her home, plan to take him for a few short visits before you go back to work. First, the two of you should be with the sitter for an hour or so just to get acquainted. Then the baby should be alone with her at a time

(Continued on the following page)

when he won't need to be fed. Then he should be with the sitter for a few longer sessions that include feeding times. Bring some familiar toys to carry the smells and thoughts of home and Mommy. Take the time to show the sitter how you want her to do things and encourage her to ask you about any problems or questions she may have. Be sure she knows how to reach you and your husband at work.

If your caregiver lives closer to your workplace than to your home, you may want to nurse your baby after you take her there in the morning and as soon as you pick her up at night. Be sure that this is acceptable to your sitter. Whether you nurse at the sitter's house or at home, one very important provision is that the sitter not feed the baby for a couple of hours before you come to pick her up so that she'll be hungry enough to nurse vigorously. It may take a few days to work out this scheduling, which is extremely important for your baby's satisfaction at the breast, for your milk supply, for your comfort, and for the success of the breastfeeding relationship.

While you may not be able to find a caregiver who has the same attitudes toward breastfeeding that you do, you do need to find one who will carry out your instructions. In other words, she can *think* the way *she* wants, as long as she *acts* the way *you* want.

offered bottles before they have fully mastered the skills of nursing at the breast develop "nipple confusion," as described in Chapter 7. They can't make the switch between the two different kinds of sucking and sometimes develop sucking problems.

It's important to strike a happy medium. Generally, introducing the bottle at about six weeks of age avoids both these problems. By this age, most babies are competent nursers and yet they're still flexible enough to try something new. Furthermore, the mother's milk supply is well established by now and flows easily enough to keep her baby happy.

If you must go back to work before this time, of course, you'll have to introduce the bottle earlier. If at all possible, though, try to hold off your return to work at least until two months postpartum, for your sake and your baby's.

While you're still home, have someone else offer a bottle

Offering the Baby the Bottle

•Have someone else give the bottles, right from the start. This is an ideal way for the baby's father to assume a larger role in his baby's care, but if this will not work out, make other arrangements. The next best bottle-feeder is the person who will care for the baby when you go back to work.

•Introduce the bottle when the baby is not frantically hungry.

•Some babies have definite preferences for one kind of nipple over another. Others don't care.

Try a contoured nipple (like the Nuk or the Kip), but just buy one or two in case your baby doesn't like it.

Be sure not to buy nipples especially made for premature infants if your baby is full-term; these nipples are made of thinner rubber, which some vigorous suckers have been known to bite pieces from and swallow.

•You may want to buy "blind" nipples, which don't have holes in them, and make your own hole with a hot pin, to ensure that the milk won't come too quickly.

To test the flow of milk, hold the bottle upside down. If milk pours out, the nipple opening is too big; if it doesn't squirt out when you squeeze the nipple with your fingers, it's too small. In the first case, there's nothing you can do other than throw the nipple out; in the second, you can make an additional hole or two.

If your baby refuses the bottle, you can try the following strategies, which sometimes work:

•Run warm water over the nipple to bring it to body temperature.

•Brush the baby's mouth with the nipple and let her grasp it herself instead of pushing it forcefully into her mouth.

•Try another style of nipple.

•Try holding the baby in another position.

•Feed the milk in a cup, an eye dropper, or a teaspoon temporarily until the baby gets the idea that food can come from a source other than the breast.

in a place *other* than the ones where you nurse most often. Some babies refuse to take a bottle from their own mothers, whose smell they associate with nursing at the breast, or in familiar nursing spots. They will, however, take a bottle from another person in another location. This someone might be the baby's father, the caregiver, or any other willing baby-feeder.

Introduce the bottle gradually, about two weeks before you plan to go back to work, so that by the time you do go back, the baby is taking one bottle-feeding every day, at the same time every day. This time should coincide with at least one of the feedings when you'll be away. While the baby is nursing on one breast, express or pump from the other breast to keep up your supply. Your baby will probably drink less milk from the bottle than she does from the breast, perhaps less than two ounces at a time. This is not a problem.

Learning How to Pump or Express Milk

If you plan to leave your own milk with your baby-sitter to give to your baby for the feedings you'll miss, the need for pumping or expressing milk is obvious. With this technique you'll be able to get milk from your breasts while you're at work, bring it home, and give it to your sitter to give to your baby the next day. You'll also be able to make extra milk that you can store in the freezer for emergencies or for unexpected feedings.

Even if you plan to use formula for missed feedings, however, pumping or expressing is an important skill to have. It can help you relieve the pressure of overfull breasts so that you feel more comfortable, it will diminish leaking, and it will help to prevent the breast infections that often result from engorgement. In the Auerbach and Guss survey mentioned earlier, 86 percent of those 567 working mothers either hand-expressed or pumped milk at missed feedings, and the women who did this tended to nurse longer.

You can't expect to do your learning when you're back on the job, pressured by time, dressed for success, and in an environment that probably provides less than ideal levels of comfort and privacy. If you start doing it at least three weeks before you go back to work, you'll be able to take time to practice and you should be fairly proficient by the time you need to be.

One technique that's especially valuable is expressing from one breast while you're nursing your baby on the other breast. This method enlists your baby as your partner, since you'll be getting the benefit of the let-down triggered by the baby's sucking and your work will be easier. You'll need help from another person the first time you try this, even if you're extremely dextrous.

If you have trouble mastering this (as many women do), try instead to pump or express some milk about an hour after a nursing while the baby is otherwise engaged. The amount you produce doesn't matter, especially in these early sessions. The point is to learn the technique.

Expressing while you're still at home will let you stockpile a supply of milk in your freezer. If you plan to feed your baby breast milk alone, you'll have a back-up supply in your freezer for emergencies and days when your supply may be low. If you plan to supplement with formula, a few extra bottles of breast milk are a happy bonus for your baby.

For step-by-step directions on both hand-expression and pumping and for a comparison of the different techniques and the different kinds of pumps, see the Appendix. You'll also find directions for storing and then using the milk that you have expressed.

BACK AT WORK

Your Work Schedule

Try to make your first day back at work a Thursday or Friday. This will give you the weekend to rest up, to analyze the way your workday went, and to see how you can help it go more smoothly.

If you can go back to work part-time for a while, this may be ideal. Survey after survey shows that mothers who work part-time seem the happiest with their lives, compared to full-time employees and full-time homemakers. This is an especially helpful arrangement, of course, for the breastfeeding mother, especially if she goes back to work before her baby is four months old.

If you have this option and can plan your schedule, fewer

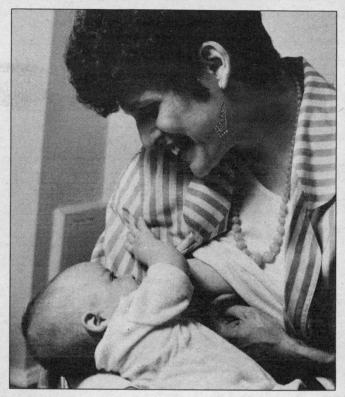

Working mothers often treasure that last nursing in the morning before they leave the baby and the first one after they return home at the end of the working day. The babies love them, too.

hours per day work out better for breastfeeding than fewer days per week. In other words, if you plan to work about 24 hours per week, you'll do better putting in five hours a day for five days instead of eight hours for three days. You'll have to balance this advantage for the nursing with any disadvantages, such as the higher expense of child care or a long commute to work, and make the decision that's best for you.

The possibilities for alternative scheduling are limitless. On some jobs you can bring some of your work home to do. On others you can take advantage of flexible scheduling or of sharing your job with another worker. At some workplaces it's possible to take your baby to work with you. Or you may be able to combine two coffee breaks into a single longer break, which you can then attach to your lunch hour so that you can go to your baby. (One mother meets her sitter, her older son, and her nursing baby in the park on sunny days and in a coffee shop on cold or rainy days.) Explore the possibility of these options with your employers. Even if they never thought of such arrangements in the past, they may be willing to give it a try.

You may decide, after adding up the costs of child care, commuting, clothes, lunches out, and so forth, that the only way for you to come out ahead is to find some work that you can do at home. Or you may be in a position to postpone your return to paid employment until your child is older.

Years ago the mother who worked outside the home was criticized for leaving her children. Today the climate has changed so far in the other direction that many women who have the financial option of staying home for a few years and who enjoy caring for small children and running a household, feel that other people consider them parasitical and useless. It would be a shame if women came to accept the judgment that a person is only as interesting and valuable as her job and her income—a way of thinking far too common among men. Bringing up children is important work, and our society needs to recognize that *every* mother is a working mother. You're the only one who can decide whether this is the sole work you want to do in these years and whether it's financially feasible for you.

Whatever your decision, if you're happy with it, your children are likely to thrive. Research has shown that the more satisfied a woman is with her life, the more effective she is as a parent, and the better adjusted her children will be.

Your Nursing Schedule

While there are as many different ways to plan your breastfeeding schedule as there are mothers and babies, a fairly typical one for a full-time mother of a small baby with fairly regular habits may go something like this:

• Wake up in the morning one hour before you need to begin to get ready for work. Take your baby back to bed with you for a quiet, leisurely feeding.

• Nurse the baby again just before you leave him at the caregiver's home or at the day care center. (Optional, depending on how much time has elapsed since the first morning feeding, and on you and your baby.)

• If you're leaving your own milk for the baby's feedings, express or pump two to three times during the work day (on morning and/or afternoon coffee breaks and/or at lunch-time).

• If feasible, nurse your baby at noon, either by going to her or having her brought to you.

• Nurse the baby right after work, at the child care site if you have a long ride home or, preferably, at home. (You will have asked the sitter not to feed the baby for a couple of hours before you're expected.)

• Nurse just before you go to sleep.

• Nurse once during the night. (Optional, depending on your baby's schedule. Many women find that getting up once during the night is not exhausting, especially if they and the baby go right back to sleep afterward.)

• Some working nursing mothers schedule "reverse cycle feeding," by which they feed their babies frequently during the evening and at night so that the babies won't be hungry during the day. Some babies seem to save their "up" time for these nighttime nursings, which are easier when mothers bring the baby into bed with them to nurse rather than awakening completely. If you can concentrate on the bonus of together time instead of the lost sleep, these snuggled-together sessions can be highlights of the nursing experience. (This schedule is described by Marilyn Grams, M.D., who used it while nursing her babies, in her book, *Breastfeeding Success for Working Mothers*.)

No one is typical, and every woman has to learn what works for her. One flight attendant, for example, went back to work after three months, making three trips a week. She chose night flights so that she would miss only one or two feedings, used a breast pump every three or four hours, put her breast milk in bottles that she packed in ice until she got home, and then froze the milk for use during her next flight. Another mother nursed full-time for her baby's first six weeks, then substituted formula for two daytime feedings a day for the next two weeks, and went back to work after two months. She continued to nurse only three times a day—morning, evening, and bedtime. Clearly, there's no single "right way." For the way one family manages, see the box on the next few pages (A Day in the Life of One Working Nursing Family).

Travel

If your job requires travel, this, of course, poses new challenges. Ideally, you'll be able to postpone any trips until your baby is weaned. If you can't, you don't necessarily have to wean because of the trip. The ingenuity of mothers and the adaptability of babies can be astonishing. You may be able to take your baby and the baby-sitter with you. If so, you might be able to maintain the same basic schedule as at home. If not, you can arrange for bottle feeding in your absence.

If you know about the trip ahead of time, you can express milk and build up a frozen supply. Or your baby can take formula in the interim. In either case, you'll want to express milk during the separation to keep up your supply and to feel comfortable. It may be possible to rent an electric pump if you'll be staying at one place for several days.

While it's sometimes possible to work out such arrangements, it's far from simple; it's to both your advantages (yours and your baby's) to make every effort to avoid this kind of separation while you're nursing.

Coworkers

Some nursing mothers find that their fellow workers, both male and female, take an interest in them and are helpful. One woman, for example, pumped her milk under a stairwell while a male colleague stood guard to protect her privacy.

A Day in the Life of One Working Nursing Family

The following schedule represents a fairly typical weekday in the life of Charlotte Lee-Carrihill, Brian Carrihill, and their children, Colin, age three, and Laura, age three months. Charlotte is an executive at a Wall Street investment banking firm; Brian is a computer graphics specialist. This family's success in handling two careers and two children, one of whom has been and the other of whom is being breastfed, rests on their willingness to work together toward common goals, support from family members who live nearby, good organization, and Charlotte's vast reserves of energy, which let her keep a very active schedule.

It's important to remember that each family needs to find its own way of doing things. This is how life works out in one household, but it might not work well in yours. You need to recognize your own and your family's unique personal needs and to plan your schedule accordingly. You may, for example, be able to sleep a little later in the morning, get to your place of work a little bit later or leave a little bit earlier, and your husband may be able to shoulder more or less of the child care duties.

Once you have your schedule worked out, you need to keep it flexible. Life has a way of interfering with the most careful plans, requiring quick changes and an acceptance that even the most ideal schedule has to be written in pencil, not ink.

6:00 A.M.	Charlotte nurses Laura, who sleeps in the same bed with her parents for the first few months of her life. If Laura doesn't wake up by herself, Charlotte wakes her up for the nursing. Brian is already awake and getting dressed.
6:15	Charlotte showers, washes her hair, dresses.
6:30	Brian leaves for work. Charlotte dresses Colin, who sleeps through the entire pro-

cess. She then dresses Laura, who has also fallen back to sleep.

7:00   Charlotte takes Colin and his lunchbox (packed the night before) out to the car. She covers him with a blanket, which she leaves in the car all the time, so the children have an easier awakening. She goes back into the house to get Laura, Laura's bag (containing diapers, an extra outfit, a bib, toys—all packed the night before, plus the day's supply of expressed milk put in at the last minute), and her own briefcase (containing cylinder-type breast pump, thermos, washcloth, a brush to clean the pump, paper towels, and nursing pads, in addition to papers she needs for work, also packed the night before).

7:10   Charlotte drops Laura off at the baby-sitter's home. (She leaves some equipment there all week, including a stroller, a walker, a quilt, a blanket, and one bottle of frozen breast milk for emergencies.)

7:25   Charlotte drops Colin off at his nursery school/day care center.

7:30   Charlotte parks her car near the subway, takes the train into work.

8–8:30   Charlotte arrives at her office. She eats breakfast either in the cafeteria with co-workers, at a breakfast meeting with clients, or alone at her desk.

10:00   Coffee break—Charlotte goes into the ladies' room where she pumps her milk and pours it into a thermos, which she'll carry home in her briefcase. She can now do both breasts in about 10 minutes.

12–12:30 P.M.   Lunch, usually at her desk, followed by a

(Continued on the following pages)

short trip outside to do errands and to get some fresh air.

1:00   Trip to the women's bathroom to pump milk.

4:00   Trip to the women's bathroom to pump milk.

5:00   Charlotte leaves her office.

5:40   Charlotte picks up Colin at school.

6:00   Brian picks up Laura at the baby-sitter's. Charlotte arrives home, gives Colin a snack to tide him over until dinner, which she starts to prepare. Over the weekend she plans the week's meals. If she gets home late or for some other reason can't hold to the original plan, she takes something out of the freezer that can be prepared quickly.

6:30   Brian and Laura arrive home. Charlotte nurses Laura. Brian brings her something to eat while she's nursing—a banana or a mini peanut butter sandwich. She also sips on a glass of ice water (which she does during most nursings). Brian continues with dinner preparations. If Charlotte has time, she takes a 15- to 20-minute run.

7:00   Brian, Charlotte, and Colin sit down to dinner. Laura is nearby in her swing or playing on a quilt on the floor.

7:30   Brian washes the dinner dishes while Charlotte puts Colin and Laura in for their baths. Brian takes Laura out of the bath and dresses her; Charlotte does the same for Colin.

8:00   Charlotte nurses Laura. She nurses her on demand all evening, every hour or two, whenever Laura seems to want to nurse. Usually this averages five or six nursings between 6 P.M. and 6 A.M. Charlotte finds this relaxing, as well as a good way to keep up her milk supply. She also nurses on demand over the weekend.

While Charlotte is nursing, Brian is playing with Colin. During the nursing, Charlotte may join in to play games, read, or watch TV with the two of them (TV is limited to one hour a day on weekdays.) Weather permitting, the four of them may go out for a walk.

8:00	(Occasionally the family goes out to dinner with family or friends. It's very rare for Charlotte and Brian to go out on weeknights without the children.)
8:30–10:00	Sometimes Charlotte throws a load of clothes into the washing machine and dryer; sometimes she does hand laundry. She always does next-day preparation: She lays out the next day's clothing for the children and herself; she makes Colin's lunch; she packs Laura's bag (except for the milk); she packs her own briefcase.
10:00	Brian gets Colin ready for bed, and Charlotte reads to him. (Because Colin takes a long nap at nursery school, he is not ready to go to sleep early. His parents are content with this schedule, since this gives them more time with him.)
10:00–10:30	Charlotte nurses Laura and puts her to bed. If she didn't run earlier, she sometimes works out now.
10:30–11:00	Brian and Charlotte have some quiet time together.
11:00	Charlotte and Brian go to sleep. They move Laura, already asleep in their bed, to her bassinet beside them.
3:00 A.M.	Charlotte nurses Laura.

Others report that their coworkers answer their phones for them while they're on their "pump breaks." Unfortunately, other mothers are targets of resentment from their colleagues, who may complain about a woman's expressing milk in an employee's lounge or bathroom or about her "getting away with" something that other workers are not.

Women handle their on-the-job relationships in various ways. Some don't tell their fellow workers what they're doing. Others go out of their way to let people know—and to show them that they are indeed doing their jobs as well as ever. One stock analyst is able to deal with the hostility she sometimes senses from the women by understanding where it comes from.

"I realize," she says, "that some of these women's resentment comes from their own pain or regrets that they didn't do this for their babies or that they're not able to be with their children as much as they would like, and I don't let their remarks bother me. I know I'm doing this because it's important for my baby, and I can't be ruled by other people's derogatory attitudes and comments. I see this as an opportunity to be a role model for some of the women in the firm who haven't had babies yet. I show them that something like this is do-able."

FEEDING YOUR BABY WHILE YOU'RE AT WORK

You need to decide long before you go back to work what your baby will drink in the bottles she receives from her caregiver. You have basically two choices—your own milk that you have expressed and pumped earlier or formula. Plain cow's milk is not an option, since current medical belief is that babies should be 12 months old before they are fed cow's milk.

Breast milk is superior in many ways to formula, for the reasons spelled out in Chapter 1. Modern formula, however, is a viable alternative, and many babies thrive beautifully on it. The one caution in introducing formula at an early age is the possibility of a baby's allergic reaction to it either now or in the future.

If you do feel that you can, as many women do, undertake and follow through on a program to express or pump milk for your baby, he can enjoy the benefits of breast milk for the entire time that you're nursing. Given your work conditions, your schedule, and your own inclinations, however, if you decide not to do this, you can substitute formula for the feedings you'll be missing. If neither you nor your husband has a family history of allergy, this is fairly safe.

If you find that you're not able to express enough milk to meet your baby's needs, you can use some formula as well. Or you may want to switch entirely to formula for the feedings while you're at work. Remember that it's better to give some breast milk than none, that worrying about the possibility of your baby's going hungry will decrease your milk output even more, and that the value of the nursing experience does not rely only on the volume of milk you produce. If you're anxious about the amount of milk you're producing, leave some formula with your sitter. It's better to do this and to be able to enjoy the emotional closeness when you do nurse than to be so anxious about the quantity of milk you're providing that neither you nor your baby will enjoy the experience.

Whichever you decide, you'll want to learn to pump or express milk, either to provide your baby's sustenance or to relieve your own discomfort. The basic instructions for expressing, pumping, storing, and giving breast milk can be found in the Appendix. We'll deal here with some special considerations for the working woman.

Expressing or Pumping Your Own Breast Milk

As we suggested earlier, you'll want to learn the techniques of expressing and/or pumping milk well before your return to work. You need to find out the method that works best for you.

Equipment You'll Need if You Decide to Pump:

•A pump that's easy to carry and store, since you'll either be taking it to work with you every day or you'll be storing it at work. If you keep it at work, you need to buy another pump to keep at home. You'll also want one that's easy to clean, especially since the washing facilities at work may not be up to the standards you have at home.

•A thermos (the kind used for fluids, not solid foods), the best

Wardrobe Tips for the Working Breastfeeding Mother

Appearance is especially important for women who face an audience of adults each day. Since you're apt to feel better about yourself and what you're doing if you're happy with the way you look, you'll want to look as good as you can, even while you're dressing for breastfeeding. These suggestions from other women may help:

•Wear breast pads in your bra for the first few weeks. They'll prevent leaking milk from coming through and showing. Be sure to change them when they get wet, to prevent sore nipples and to avoid the possibility of moisture showing through. (See Chapter 5 for suggestions.)

•Wear bright or dark print blouses or tops. They won't show any leaking that does occur as readily as solids and they won't show the outlines of your nipples or your breast pads. Stay away from whites and pale colors; they reveal to everyone what you may just want your baby and your husband to see.

•Cottons and synthetic fabrics stand up best in case of leaking. Silks and linens may be stained. Clinging materials will show the outlines of nipples and breast pads.

•Everything you wear should be washable. Nothing should need more than touch-up ironing.

•If you're self-conscious about your more bosomy figure,

quality you can find. Before you leave home in the morning fill it with ice cubes to keep it cold. When you express, dump out the ice and fill the thermos with your milk.

•A photo of your baby, to prop in front of you while you express. Some mothers find that this helps trigger their letdown.

•A brush for cleaning the pump after each use.

wear a lightweight blazer or loose jacket during your workday.

•Don't try to squeeze into too-tight prepregnancy clothes. Chances are that you're a few pounds heavier than you were then, and clothes that strain are unbecoming to even the slimmest women. Try wearing what you wore to work early in your pregnancy before you put on maternity clothes.

•Tight blouses are especially treacherous since they rub against your nipples and might trigger a let-down at the most inconvenient times, like on the subway or in an important meeting.

•Keep a spare blouse at work (one that can be worn with most outfits) in case you leak or spill milk on the one you're wearing.

If you're expressing milk or nursing your baby during the workday:

•Wear a nursing bra to work. It's more convenient to be able to undo one side at a time instead of having to take off your entire bra. You'll also welcome its support.

•Wear blouses or tops with skirts or pants.

•Avoid dresses and jumpsuits and blouses that button down the back.

•Wear blouses or tops that button down the front or pull up easily. Don't wear cotton sweaters; they tend to lose their shape during the day after being pulled up two or three times.

•A washcloth for patting your breasts dry after expressing. (Do not wipe; wiping removes natural oil secretions and can cause chapping and soreness.)

•A cloth or paper towels for wiping the rim of the thermos and the pump.

•An extra set of nursing pads.

•A bag or briefcase, in which you can carry the equipment between work and home in separate plastic bags.

Where to Express. Try to find a clean, quiet, private place. Ideally, a quiet office with a door, either your own office or another that you can arrange to use, is best. A vacant meeting or conference room may be available. Many women use a women's lounge or bathroom. One confessed to a special fondness for the stall in her bathroom designed for handicapped women, since it's roomier and has a convenient shelf for placing her paraphernalia.

When to Express. At first it may take you up to 30 minutes each session to empty both breasts; eventually you may be able to get it down to eight minutes each time; some women continue to need 15 to 20 minutes. The more you practice at home, the better you'll do.

You should be able to find enough time between your coffee breaks and your lunch hour. In your eagerness to make the most of the time, however, don't neglect your diet. You need to keep your strength up. You may be able to take your lunch at your desk. If you can't get enough time during your breaks, you may be able to make arrangements to come in earlier, stay later, or take work home. Or you may be so efficient that you do your job in less time.

How Much to Express. At first you may not get more than an ounce at a time, but eventually you can probably count on expressing three to five ounces of milk at each session. You'll most likely produce more milk early in the day and early in the week. If you can't get enough for your baby's next-day feedings, try some of the hints given on page 152 or the Appendix. It's still worth pumping even if you get just one ounce from each side, since you can mix your milk with formula. When you're at home, evenings and weekends, nurse the baby on demand, or even more frequently than the baby requests. This will help you increase your milk supply. Don't give any bottles at all when you're home. If you express during some of these nursings, you can accumulate extra stores of milk.

How to Handle the Expressed Milk. As soon as you get home, pour the milk from the thermos into clean four-ounce plastic bottles. The bottles don't need to be sterilized if the milk has been kept cold, but they do need to be washed thoroughly to be sure that no milk particles are left. Rinse them out, swish a bottle brush around the inside, including the rim, and then wash in hot, soapy water. Rinse well. If you have a dishwasher, wash them in there.

In the first six hours after expression, human milk kept in a capped clean container does not grow bacteria, even at room temperature. This means that even if you are not able to keep your milk refrigerated or on ice, you can still collect it. If you cannot refrigerate the milk, however, it is safer to store it in a sterile container. Cap it tightly, keep it out of the sun and away from heating units, and refrigerate the milk as soon as you get home. It will be ready to take the next day to your sitter packed in ice or blue ice-packs in a cooler. If you have more milk than you'll need right away, put it in a freezer.

You can freeze your milk directly in the plastic bottle. The four-ounce size is best so that you can defrost small amounts. If your freezer maintains a temperature of $0°$ F, the milk will keep for months. (You can check this with a freezer thermometer.) Try to keep an extra emergency stock in the freezer so you won't get nervous about running out. You can do this by expressing during nursings at home.

Instead of pumping into a thermos, some women do it into a wide-mouthed jar and then pour the milk into a bottle. They then store it among ice cubes or ice-packs in a thermos jug or small cooler. The method works fine. The disadvantage is that it involves carrying bulkier equipment. Some women like the disposable bottle bags that come in nurser kits because they lie flat in a freezer, are easy to stack, and thaw quickly. Others find them hard to handle and easy to puncture. You have to find out what works best for you.

Be prepared for the unexpected, which will always happen. If you're ingenious and creative, you'll be able to handle whatever comes up. One mother dropped and broke her thermos of the day's expressed milk—and saved the next day by going home and expressing while she nursed that evening and the next morning. Her baby was already sleeping through the night, so the mother set her alarm to wake herself up every three hours all night long to express enough milk for the following day. Thanks to the law of supply and demand, her breasts responded to the frequent stimulation.

Formula

If you plan to offer formula to your baby, you'll have to replace one or more breastfeedings with formula feedings. This change must be done gradually, to avoid engorgement and the risk of breast infection. You'll need to allow between four and seven days per feeding, or more, if you're eliminating breastfeedings that will be replaced by exclusive bottle-feedings. Even pumping produces some nipple stimulation and therefore some milk. As you begin to substitute the formula for your own milk, you may need to express manually to relieve your discomfort. If so, save your milk. You can use it for the baby, providing a switch by substituting breast milk occasionally for formula.

On weekends and holidays, you can maintain your weekday schedule, except for one additional breastfeeding. This keeps your milk supply at a fairly constant, comfortable level. Again, you'll want someone else to give those bottles to your baby, since he may not accept them from you.

Working mothers are like other breastfeeding mothers in citing their biggest problem as fatigue. Since it's especially hard for you to get the rest you need, you have to be ruthless in cutting out everything in your life that is not absolutely essential. Doing your work and taking care of your family should be the only things you have to worry about for the time that you're nursing. This is the time to cut back and to enjoy this precious time of your life, so that you can look back in later years to many happy memories of this special shared experience. As one breastfeeding working mother says, "It lasts for such a tiny part of the children's lives that it needs to be cherished."

10

Breastfeeding: A Sexual Passage

The months following the birth of a first child constitute a difficult period of time in every marriage. As with any other new experience, you are likely to welcome parenthood with mixed emotions. The birth of your first baby brings home to you and your husband more dramatically than any other event in your lives the realization that you are no longer children but are now adults, newly responsible for another human being. Eager as you may be to grow into this phase of life, it's only natural that you would feel anxious about what it will mean and what will be expected of you. If you and your husband have been able to communicate well before the arrival of the baby, you will have a good base to help you adjust to parenthood. If not, it's especially important for you to make extra efforts now to let each other know exactly how you feel.

Like every other woman in the world, you have to learn to be a mother. It does not happen magically via labor and delivery. You need time and practice to feel at home in your new role. Meanwhile, you are likely to worry about your ability to be a good mother, and your husband has his own conflicts to struggle with as he faces up to the responsibility of parenthood. Yet all too often, both husband and wife will assume that their partners know how they feel, and neither one expresses his or her real concerns.

The experience of breastfeeding introduces other elements into this period of your life, since as a lactating woman, you are experiencing a powerful phase in the female cycle of sexuality. The physiological changes that occur in your body in connection with pregnancy, childbirth, and lactation are likely to affect your emotions, your sexual desires, and your relationship with your man. Breastfeeding dramatizes the physical and emotional ties in the new couple (you and your child) that overlap with those in the preexisting couple (you and your husband). Furthermore, both you and your husband are bound to respond in some way to those cultural signals in our society that accentuate the sexual symbolism of the breasts.

Different women respond differently to this aspect of their reproductive and sexual functioning, with some finding that breastfeeding enhances their sense of themselves as sexual beings and others feeling that it seems to relegate their sexuality to the "back burner." Before we talk about concerns revolving around the intimacy of the husband-wife relationship and the impact of breastfeeding on your sexuality, let's look at some of the ways in which breastfeeding serves as a sexual passage in both of your lives.

FEMALE SEXUALITY

Historically, the dominant thread in discussions of sexuality has consisted of allusions to sexual intercourse. People have been considered fulfilled sexual beings if they have been able to reach orgasm through intercourse. This definition has often focused on men, either ignoring women's needs for sexual gratification or assuming that they should achieve such gratification in the same way men did, through intercourse. In recent years, however, largely due to the impact of the women's movement, the distinctly female sexual experience has gained greater recognition. One benefit of this recognition has been the development of a more global definition of sexuality, keying it more into sensuality and to the many pleasurable sensations that can be reached through a wide range of activities, which may include, but are not limited to, sexual intercourse. By thinking of sexuality in this way, we expand the possibility of sexual fulfillment to include times in life when intercourse may not be possible, advisable, or desirable, such as the weeks just before and just after the birth of a baby.

Both men and women can and do derive great pleasure from such noncoital activities as kissing, stroking, touching, cuddling, massage, and various kinds of oral and manual stimulation. In addition, women's sexuality is even more wideranging, closely tied in as it is to the five phases in their reproductive capacity, consisting of the menstrual cycle, orgasm from direct sexual stimulation, pregnancy, childbirth, and lactation.

All five of these phases are controlled to a large measure by the interaction of many of the hormones released inside a woman's body. Estrogen, progesterone, testosterone, folliclestimulating hormone (FSH), luteinizing hormone (LH), oxytocin, and prolactin are among the hormones that help to make a woman a sexual being. Some of these substances manage the course of the menstrual cycle, causing ovulation and subsequently fertility. Some dominate during pregnancy. Others signal the onset of labor, the production and release of milk, and the climax of orgasm. Most of these hormones have more than one function. While some are more active during one phase of the female cycle than are others, the interaction among them is responsible for some remarkable similarities in the various sexual phases, as shown in the box on the next page (The Interrelationships Among the Five Phases of Female Sexuality).

Female sexuality, then, involves a complex series of responses that carry over from a woman's reproductive capacity to her maternal functions. Yet in our society, woman's interest in sexual intercourse—in achieving her own orgasm and in helping her man to achieve his—has been stressed, while those elements of sexuality related to childbirth and lactation have been virtually ignored. Dr. Alice Rossi, a sociology professor at the University of Massachusetts, has suggested that our "male dominant family and political systems have imposed a wedge between maternalism on the one hand, and female sexuality on the other. We define maternity in culturally narrow ways, clearly differentiate it from sexuality, and require that women deny the evidence of their senses by repressing the component of sexuality in the maternal role."

The Interrelationships Among the Five Phases of Female Sexuality

HOW OUTSIDE PRESSURES AND EMOTIONS CAN INFLUENCE ALL FIVE PHASES

•*The Menstrual Cycle:* The most regular *cycle* can be disrupted by excitement or anxiety. A bride, for example, may have carefully set the date for her marriage—and yet still menstruate on her wedding day. Or the tension of a job or family crisis may bring on or suspend a woman's menses.

•*Orgasm from Sexual Stimulation:* The tremendous impact of outside influences on *sexual interaction* is obvious to anyone (male *or* female) who can't get in the mood for sex because of the distractions of financial, family, job, or health problems. Or a woman at the brink of orgasm may be abruptly "turned off" by a piercing yell from the nursery, by the ringing of the telephone, or by a fear that her privacy is about to be invaded.

•*Pregnancy:* Conception itself may be affected by emotional influences. Studies in animal and human reproduction suggest that stress may affect hormone production in a way that interferes with ovulation.

•*Childbirth:* Outside events also influence childbirth. An emotional or physical shock can bring on premature labor, and the mother's anticipation of childbirth often seems related to the ease and duration of labor and delivery. The woman who is frightened of giving birth is apt to have a

This attitude, fortunately, is being overcome, partly due to the women's movement and partly due to greater acceptance of sexuality in general. The work of sex researchers William H. Masters and Virginia E. Johnson, for example, has had an enormous influence on the ways in which people think more difficult delivery than the woman who understands the physiology of childbirth.

•*Lactation:* Mothers and midwives have long known that a woman's ability to give milk to her baby is influenced by such factors as pain, embarrassment, or emotional conflict. Doctors Michael and Niles Newton confirmed this observation in the laboratory, showing that a successfully nursing mother will give significantly less milk when she is distracted during feedings by annoyances and pain.

OTHER PHENOMENA COMMON TO MORE THAN ONE PHASE OF FEMALE SEXUALITY

•*The breasts enlarge* just before menstruation, during pregnancy, just before orgasm, and during lactation.

•*The nipples become erect* upon sexual stimulation, during childbirth, and during lactation.

•*The uterus contracts* during orgasm, childbirth, and lactation.

•*Body temperature rises* during ovulation, childbirth, orgasm, and lactation.

•*A woman usually feels an urge to take care of her loved one* in a fulfilling sexual relationship, during pregnancy, after childbirth, and during lactation.

•*The hormone oxytocin surges through a woman's body* during orgasm, during childbirth, and during lactation. This hormone causes the uterus to contract and the nipples to become erect. Oxytocin is also the stimulus for the milk-ejection reflex and probably the reason why milk sometimes spurts from the breasts of a woman in orgasm.

about sex. In recent years we have learned a great deal about the actual physiological mechanisms related to sexual activities and responses. We have felt freer to communicate with our sexual partners about how we feel and what we like, and many couples have found that their sexual rapport flourishes in such an open climate. The same can happen when we are open and understanding about aspects of sexuality in the maternal role.

THE SENSUOUS NATURE OF BREASTFEEDING

In *Human Sexual Response*, the 1966 book that reported on their pioneering research, Masters and Johnson included the results of interviews with 111 women during and after their pregnancies. These women talked about their sexual behavior, feelings, and responses during pregnancy and immediately following childbirth. Of this group, only 24 women nursed their babies (a reflection of the low popularity of breastfeeding when this research was done).

Some of these nursing mothers reported experiencing sexual arousal while suckling their babies. Several said that they felt guilty about this and worried that they were "perverted." Some women who did not breastfeed said they were afraid that they might be sexually stimulated from the suckling.

Three of the women in the Masters and Johnson study reported incidents of orgasm while nursing, although this seems rare among the general population. Other researchers have found that nursing mothers are more likely to report a sense of satisfaction similar to the euphoria that follows orgasm rather than the intensity and excitement of the orgasm itself. Women most often talk about a calm feeling of completion that combines physical and emotional fulfillment. In her book *Free and Female*, Barbara Seaman describes nursing as "a sensual and sensuous experience unlike any other, somewhat related to and yet different from good sex."

It shouldn't be surprising that breastfeeding has its sensual components. For many women, the breasts are highly erogenous zones, sensitive to the slightest touch and capable of sending messages of excitation throughout the body. In fact, some women reach orgasm from having their breasts fondled. The nerve pathways from the nipple to the brain are the same, no matter what the stimulation is. During lactation, of course, the breasts are constantly stimulated both by the mother's own handling and by the baby's extensive sucking and sometimes frequent stroking.

Furthermore, our society has eroticized the breast even beyond its own intrinsic nature, and most nursing mothers are very conscious of their breasts as sexual symbols as well as sources of nutrition and comfort for their babies. (This, of course, is why so many women are reluctant to expose their breasts in public. Even if they don't see the act as sexually provocative, they know that there are others who will.)

Unfortunately, many women who experience sexual arousal while nursing their babies are apt to feel guilty—so guilty that they may wean their babies early and refuse to nurse future children. In our society sexual feelings are supposed to stay in their place—to come out of hiding only when a culturally determined suitable partner is present. Yet we are sexual beings, and our sexual feelings spin a thread that runs through the fabric of our entire lives.

Many women do, of course, appreciate the sensuous nature of breastfeeding. They realize that nursing is supposed to be enjoyable for both mother and baby. If it were not, our species could never have survived the thousands of years when no substitute for human milk was available. Some researchers have concluded that when women are encouraged to accept and enjoy the sexual pleasure breastfeeding can offer, they give more milk. This makes sense, since the let-down reflex is highly subject to emotional influences. Indeed, the good feelings associated with breastfeeding may be built into our natures to strengthen the bond between mother and baby in the early months of life.

Not all women experience sexual sensations from breastfeeding, and those who don't needn't feel that they are repressed or inhibited. They simply have a different experience. In his landmark book, *Sexual Behavior in the Human Female,* Dr. Alfred E. Kinsey stated that only half of all women seem to derive any satisfaction from having their breasts fondled—and that both oral and manual stimulation of the female breasts are often more exciting to the man who touches than to the woman who is touched. A woman whose breasts are not normally erogenous is not likely to become erotically stimulated by the suckling of her infant. And even a woman whose breasts ordinarily respond to her husband's touch or kiss may find that during lactation, they become almost insensitive to touch—his as well as his baby's.

Also, it's been said many times that the most powerful sex organ in the human body is the brain. Situations that we think about as sexual are more arousing than those that we don't imbue with sexual connotations. Thus, a woman may be concentrating so fully on feeding and interacting with her baby that she is not even aware of physical sensations that in other circumstances might be very erotic.

In sum, there is no right or wrong way for your body to respond sexually to the nursing experience. You can be a successful nursing mother if you do become erotically aroused by breastfeeding—or if such feelings are the farthest thing from your mind.

HOW NURSING MOTHERS FEEL ABOUT SEX

"There is something very earthy about nursing a child that can pleasantly affect the husband-wife relationship. And I also feel that a good breastfeeding experience makes you more open and womanly. Because of nursing . . . I was able to have orgasms which I had never had before."

"I'm sure that nursing had something to do with my lack of interest in sex. My body was in use all day long. I felt as if somebody was constantly sucking on me and holding me and being held by me, and by the time night came around I just wanted to draw an invisible circle around my body and say, 'No trespassing.'"

Two different women—both breastfeeding, both in good marriages, each with a totally different attitude about sex. Both of them are normal, and both have plenty of company. Nursing mothers seem to fall about equally into two distinct camps. Some, like the first woman quoted, experience increased sexual appetites and enjoy a much less sexually inhibited relationship with their husbands. Other women find that they are not nearly as interested in sex for the first six months after childbirth as they had been before or will be again.

A number of studies, starting with Masters and Johnson's, have found that, in general, breastfeeding women resume sexual activity sooner after childbirth than do bottle-feeding mothers and that nursing and sexuality are positively related.

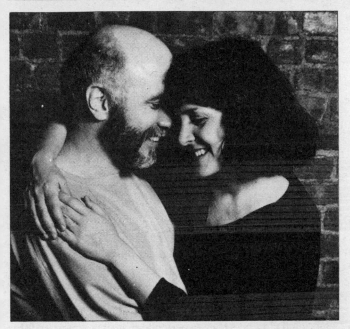

Time for affection is still important after lovers become parents.

In Dr. Alice K. Ladas's survey of more than 1,000 nursing mothers, 30 percent of the women reported that their sexual relationships with their husbands had improved after nursing, while only 2.5 percent reported worsened relationships. Most of the women who said they now had a better sex life had considered their sexual relationship excellent before nursing, while all the women in the other category said they had had a poor sexual adjustment to begin with.

Women who feel sexier while nursing might be particularly sensuous and more comfortable with their bodies than the average woman. They may have fewer feelings of embarrassment about handling or exposing their breasts. They may even welcome the opportunity to breastfeed as a chance to experience a new kind of bodily sensation. They may be more sensitive to physical sensations and more accepting of body secretions. They may have especially erogenous breasts that respond to the constant stimulation of the baby's suckling. Or they may have especially high stores of oxytocin in their system. While this potent chemical is contributing to their success in nursing, it may also produce increased levels of eroticism. One mother has said, "Of course I didn't always feel sexy when I was nursing the baby—which is a good thing while I was feeding her ten times a day!—but sometimes the combination of nursing her and seeing my husband in bed next to me made me want to rush through the feeding so that Bob and I could make love."

On the other hand, there are many factors that can diminish a nursing woman's interest in sex. One that affects most new mothers whether they nurse or not is fatigue. Taking care of a baby is hard work. Furthermore, the new mother must adjust to the constant interruption of her sleep. Add to this a first-time mother's concern about her ability to care for her new baby, and it's easy to understand some women's temporarily diminished interest in lovemaking.

The "touched-out" feeling expressed by the second woman quoted earlier is fairly common. Many nursing mothers immerse themselves so deeply into their babies' care and derive so much pleasure from the physical as well as the emotional closeness they experience that they don't need this kind of closeness with their men. In fact, they sometimes need the opposite—a time when they can pull into themselves like turtles in a shell, and "reclaim" their bodies for themselves.

Furthermore, female physiology seems to discourage sexual activity in the nursing mother: Because of her lower levels of estrogen (caused by the higher levels of prolactin in her body during lactation), her vaginal wall becomes thinner and more sensitive and vaginal lubrication is reduced. Many women find that their nipples and breasts are less sensitive to touch while they're lactating. Some women also find that their nipples lose their ability to become erect on stimulation, even though they still become elongated in the baby's mouth. These responses may be nature's way of discouraging another pregnancy too soon.

Men and women generally have different attitudes toward sex during pregnancy and after childbirth. While there are situations in which the woman is more sexually eager than the man, the more common situation is for the man to press for a resumption of sexual relations, especially intercourse, while the woman is content without it. Some researchers suggest that women can accept the disruptions in their sexual relationships more easily than men do, that they're more apt to dismiss the impact of child rearing as a temporary sexual inconvenience, while men seem more likely to feel that children interfere with sex. How much of this is physical and how much cultural is hard to determine, but there are some obvious physical reasons.

A man's body does not, of course, undergo the changes that a woman's does. His shape does not change; he is not uncomfortable in various positions; he is not exhausted and sore after childbirth. Nor do the hormones in his body change radically during pregnancy and after childbirth. All of these physiological differences affect women in various ways, one of which is often a reduced desire for sex. Furthermore, men often find emotional comfort in sex, while many women are comforted more by being held and caressed. Still, women who may not be hungry for sex themselves will often be ready to resume relations because they want to give of themselves to their husbands.

No matter which camp you fall into, whether you're eager to resume sexual relations or just willing to go along for your husband's sake, you probably have many questions about lovemaking. You wonder how soon you should go back to enjoying regular sexual relations—and whether you should restrict your activities in any way, for your own sake or for your baby's.

WHAT NURSING MOTHERS DO ABOUT SEX

Most doctors advise women not to engage in sexual intercourse until after their postpartum examination. This is to prevent the two biggest postpartum risks, infection and hemorrhage, either of which can result from the introduction of an object into the vagina before it is fully healed from childbirth. Before a new mother is ready for intercourse, she should be sure that any vaginal tears or episiotomy incisions have healed, that the tenderness in her perineal area is less severe, that the placental site (the place on the uterus where the placenta had been attached until it was sheared away during childbirth) has healed, and that her vaginal canal has again developed the microorganisms that protect it from infection. (Generally, once soreness has gone, stitches have healed, and bleeding has stopped, intercourse is safe.)

This postpartum exam may take place anywhere from two to six weeks after delivery, depending on an individual doctor's general policy and sometimes on an individual patient's desires. If you want an earlier postpartum exam than your doctor customarily schedules, ask whether this is possible. It's also a good idea to ask your doctor to explain to both you and your husband together the reasons for the abstinence before this exam. Men who understand these reasons are less likely to pressure their wives to resume intercourse before the women are ready.

Sexual intercourse is not, of course, the only way by which a man and woman can keep their sexual relationship alive. You can enjoy physical, sensual closeness in many other ways, even when intercourse is not medically appropriate or desirable. You can, for example, bathe together and be nude in bed together. You can caress and fondle and stroke and massage each other. You can satisfy each other sexually through oral or manual alternatives to intercourse.

When you do resume sexual intercourse, you may find that you're still tender in the perineal area and intercourse may be painful. If you had a cesarean birth, you may experience abdominal discomfort (as well as vaginal pain if you had an unexpected cesarean after a difficult labor). This is common and is almost always only temporary. Your discomfort can be alleviated by going slowly, allowing manual or oral stimulation first until you are ready for penile penetration. It may also be helpful to use a vaginal lubricant (like K-Y jelly, Lubrin inserts, or contraceptive jelly) and a position that allows the woman to control the depth of penetration, such as the female-superior or side-by-side positions. If pain persists for seven to 10 days after resuming intercourse, call your doctor. You should feel good after having had a baby; if you're not, your pain may signal a medical problem.

If you began doing Kegel exercises soon after delivery, your enjoyment of intercourse is likely to be enhanced. These exercises speed healing, minimize pain and swelling, and strengthen the perineal muscles. To do them, you contract and relax the group of muscles directly between your legs that involve the urethra, the vagina, and to a lesser extent, the anus. The exercise routine consists of alternating a contraction of your muscles as if you are holding back the flow of urine, with the relaxation of these muscles.

If any activities or positions are painful for you now, let your husband know. Being a martyr won't feel good for you—or him. He'll sense your lack of enthusiasm for sex and may attribute it to problems in your feelings for him rather than your physical feelings. Besides, as you let him know what does not feel good, you can also take the opportunity to show him what *does* feel good.

Many nursing mothers wonder whether the breasts belong to the baby during lactation and should be off-limits to the baby's father. They need not be. You can be your husband's sexual partner during the time you are nursing your baby, and you can share your breasts with both baby and husband. Your breasts do not have to stop performing their erotic function just because they are now performing their biological function.

There is no reason why your husband cannot stimulate your breasts both manually and orally during the time you are nursing, if this is enjoyable to you. In fact, oral and manual manipulation by the husband of his wife's breasts during both pregnancy and lactation may even help to prevent sore nipples. Furthermore, your husband won't be stealing candy from his baby if he gets an occasional swallow of your good milk. There is plenty more where that came from, and as you remember from Chapter 6, the more milk that is removed from the breasts, the more will be produced.

You may find, particularly in the first couple of months, that your breasts become hard and tender an hour or two after a feeding. At these times, intercourse in the male-superior position is apt to be uncomfortable. You would probably be more comfortable in such positions as the female-superior, side-by-side, or rear-entry. This might be the perfect time to experiment with other lovemaking positions that you have never tried. You may even discover something you like better than your former favorites. In any case, the tenderness of the newly lactating breast goes away soon. After a couple of months, it will not be a factor in how you do what you do.

One woman told us, "When Joe and I first realized that every time I experienced orgasm my breasts would spurt milk, it was a big source of satisfaction for both of us. There was no doubt in his mind that I had reached a climax, and I loved being able to show it in one more way."

Spurting of milk during and immediately after orgasm is fairly common among nursing women, with the milk usually flowing more slowly from the breast that has been suckled more recently. While many women feel happy about this show of excitement, those who want to avoid spots on the sheet find that making love right after a feeding helps. It's also possible to wear a bra during sex. (There are some very appealing lacy nursing bras.)

BIRTH CONTROL

Nursing mothers are less likely to become pregnant than women who are not fully lactating. Based on records in societies where long-term nursing is the rule and on studies of nursing, partially nursing, and bottle-feeding mothers in this country, we can point to considerable evidence that breastfeeding postpones pregnancy. However, lactation is in no way a fool-proof method of contraception.

Generally, if your nursing baby is receiving no supplemental bottles or solid food and is being nursed during the night as well as during the day, the hormonal balance in your body will prevent ovulation and therefore pregnancy for three to six months or longer. Generally, you will have one "sterile" menstrual period before you begin to ovulate. But you cannot depend on it. Women have become pregnant while fully lactating and before their menses have resumed. Some women have discovered their pregnancies at the six-week postpartum exam. Women who do not want to conceive right away need to use some form of contraception.

Some kinds of birth control are more suitable than others during lactation, as shown in the box on the facing page (Contraception for the Nursing Mother). As in so many personal decisions, each of us has to weigh the pros and cons of each choice and decide upon the method that best suits our own

Contraception for the Nursing Mother

RECOMMENDED	REASONING
Diaphragm	Safe, with no side effects for mother or baby, except for very small risk of toxic shock syndrome. Up to 98 percent effective[1] if used properly and consistently, with spermicidal jelly or cream (which also provide lubrication). You must be refitted after each birth.
Sponge	Believed to have no side effects for mother or baby, except for very small risk of toxic shock syndrome (especially if left in vagina more than 24 hours), but since it does contain various chemicals and has not been researched extensively, should not be used immediately postpartum without a doctor's approval. Eighty to 90 percent effective.
Condom	Safe, with no side effects. It must be put on before any semen is expelled from penis and must be removed after ejaculation to prevent slipping off when erection subsides. Ninety percent effective. Even more effective when used in combination with spermicide.

[1]Effectiveness rates are from *Contraceptive Technology 1984–1985* (1984), a handbook for medical practitioners by Robert A. Hatcher et al. (Irvington Publications), and are the typical ones reported for each method.

(Continued on the next page)

Spermicidal Foam, Jelly, Cream, or Suppository	Eighty-two percent effective (more so when used in combination with a condom), provides lubrication (sometimes to the point of messiness). Must be used before each act of intercourse. Some women allergic.
Sterilization	Female sterilization can often be performed at time of delivery. Male sterilization can be performed at any time. Both should be regarded as irreversible. If you are absolutely sure that you do not want any more children, either you or your husband can choose surgical sterilization, today the most common form of birth control in this country.
NOT RECOMMENDED	**REASONING**
Birth Control Pills	The hormones in the combination estrogen-progestin pill often inhibit the production of milk. The progestin-only "minipill" has a higher failure rate and higher rates of break-through bleeding. The hormones in both kinds pass through the milk to the baby, and we don't know the possible long-term effects of daily doses of estrogen and progesterone on an infant's developing endocrine system.
IUDs (Intrauterine Devices)	Recent studies indicate that lactating women are 10 times more likely to experience perforation of the uterus or other problems from IUDs, possibly because their uter-

(Continued on the next page)

	ine walls are thinner due to their lower levels of estrogen. IUDs are not widely available anymore.
Natural Family Planning	Cannot be relied upon until menses are regular, which rarely happens during lactation.
Coitus Interruptus (Withdrawal)	Very unreliable in preventing pregnancy. Sexually unfulfilling for both partners.
Abstinence	While this is the only method that is 100 percent effective, it's the least suited to a satisfying relationship.

physiology, personality, and life-styles—as well as those of our partners.

If you have been taking birth control pills or wearing an IUD, it may be hard to adjust to one of the barrier methods (diaphragm, sponge, spermicide, and/or condom), the use of which is closely tied to the specific time of intercourse. While this may at first seem intrusive and a nuisance, many couples have found that they can make inserting the diaphragm or putting on the condom part of their sexual foreplay and that doing it together is an act of shared love and responsibility.

YOUR HUSBAND IS STILL YOUR LOVER

As we said before, this is a trying time in the life of a marriage. You, for example, may suddenly find, as you struggle in the morass of diapers and colic and nursing, that you would like to be a little girl again and have someone else care for you and your baby. Meanwhile, your husband, who is awed by the competent way you feed, bathe, and diaper the baby, sees only your outer shell of self-assurance. You may seem so capable in carrying out your maternal responsibilities and so self-sufficient as a nursing mother, that he underestimates your need for him. He may feel left out of the tight little circle around you and your baby.

At the same time, this new responsibility of caring for a baby often reawakens a new father's own dependency needs. One study found that expectant fathers' heightened needs for mothering showed up in an increased frequency of phone calls and letters to their own parents and requests for stories about their own birth and infancy. At this time your husband needs your reassurance that he has not slipped to second place in your life. While he recognizes intellectually that the baby requires a great deal of your time and energy, he may not be able to help resenting all the attention lavished on the newborn—attention that was formerly his alone. In addition, he sees you sharing with the baby not only your time, energy, attention, and affection, but also the breasts that were formerly revealed only to him. Is it any wonder that he should be a little jealous of his own baby?

Such feelings are natural, but many husbands are ashamed of feeling this way and will not admit them. Others express them quite openly. Aware that your husband may feel this way, you can show him that he is still the most important man in your life and that your love for him has not diminished because of your love for his baby. There are many ways you can do this. It's hard to have to think of one more thing at a time when you're facing so many new demands, but it's important to make extra efforts to preserve and enhance your relationship with your husband. You can adjust to being a mother without forgetting that you are still a wife. The suggestions in the box on the facing page (Keeping Romance in Your Marriage) might help you both over some rough spots.

One of the most important things you can do for your children is to bring your husband into the family circle as early as possible. This decision can help them forge a close relationship with their father and can help them feel good about themselves throughout their lives. If he's interested in doing things for his baby, don't limit him to fetching and carrying. Encourage him to hold, play with, and bathe the baby. If, like some men, your husband is not terribly interested in doing a great deal with the young infant, it's probably better not to

Keeping Romance in Your Marriage

•Disruptions of the dinner hour seem to hit some men harder than anything else. You can minimize these by waiting to prepare dinner until right after a feeding. Then if you and your husband pitch in together, you might be able to cook and eat dinner before the baby needs you again. No matter how much of a gourmet you may have been before the birth of the baby, be prepared for drastic changes in your eating habits, at least for the first few months when the baby's schedule is apt to be irregular. The best kind of meal for this time is one that takes a minimum amount of preparation, such as a casserole that can be put together whenever one of you has time, fish that can be broiled quickly, or a salad or stew that won't mind waiting. If you have access to good, nutritious take-out food and can afford the extra expense (along with paper plates), this is the time to splurge.

•The simplest meal can take on a romantic aura if you eat by candlelight and accompany it with a little wine.

•If you're used to having an occasional drink before dinner with your husband, you don't need to give it up. You can enjoy a glass of wine while you're nursing the baby and catching up with your husband on the day's events (both his and yours). This will provide a quiet interlude for the two of you—and may even help your milk to flow more freely.

•Make at-home dates ahead of time with your husband. These are evenings when you're not available for company, when you turn the ring off your telephone or take it off the hook, and when you set aside time just for each other. You need this relaxed time together, whether you use it for talking, for a relaxing massage or hot bath, or for an evening of watching a special TV show or videocassette. (A videocassette recorder is a wonderful gift if the proud grandparents want to give you something extravagant.)

These evenings at home can also, of course, be wonderful times for making love. While planning ahead for

(Continued on the following pages)

lovemaking may seem unromantic at first, it's worth noting that in our society marriage is the only structure that demands spontaneous sex. Dating couples and extramarital lovers *know* they have to plan ahead to see each other—and they usually find the planning itself erotic. Married couples can have an "affair" with each other, too.

•Be flexible. Even if you've usually made love before you went to sleep at night, planning your day differently now may help you get together more happily. Some couples, for example, now make love in the early morning after the baby's first nursing of the day. Some husbands are able to get home for lunch at a time when their babies conveniently take a nap. And one husband who had felt ignored because his wife was always asleep by the time he would get into bed with her after the 11 o'clock news finally realized that he could get into bed with her at about 8:30, snuggle for a while, make love, and then, after she went to sleep, he could get out of bed to watch the news.

•Even though you are nursing, you can still leave your baby for a few hours at a time. Many couples plan an evening out once a week, so that they can enjoy each other's company in a more carefree way. This need not be anything elaborate—maybe just a trip to a movie or a nearby ice cream parlor. It's best if you can plan to go out at a time when your baby usually sleeps, but if there is no "usually," you can nurse the baby just before you leave and then leave him or her with a competent sitter—possibly a student nurse, an older woman, or a college student. Once your milk supply is well established (usually by the end of the second month), you should be able to be away from the baby during feeding-time by leaving a bottle that contains your own milk, which you've either hand-expressed or pumped earlier in the day.

push him, but to wait for his attitude to change—as it probably will the first time his baby smiles at him.

If you are with a man you love, you're lucky, indeed. You have the opportunity to give of yourself and to be physically

While you and your husband are renewing your relationship, your baby can be learning to trust other people besides the two of you. As the noted anthropologist Margaret Mead used to say, babies are most likely to develop into well-adjusted human beings when they are cared for "by many warm, friendly people"—as long as most of these loved people remain in the infants' lives.

•If your baby sleeps in the same bed with you, you need to realize that bed is not the only place where lovemaking can take place. Why else was the rug in front of the fireplace invented?

•Pay attention to yourself. Your baby will think you're beautiful no matter what, but you'll feel better about yourself and show your husband that you care about his opinion if you can do some minimal grooming feats shortly before you expect him home, like running a comb through your hair and putting on a blouse that doesn't have that unmistakable perfume of spit-up milk. Women who are ordinarily small-breasted sometimes enjoy dressing seductively during the time they're nursing, when they're more bosomy than they ever have been before. Women who are less thrilled about their added pounds and curves can feel and look more attractive if they buy one or two appealing outfits (as suggested in Chapter 5).

•If you're eager to resume sexual relations with your husband, don't be shy about letting him know. He may be waiting for a signal from you. If you couldn't care less, you may want to go along to meet his needs. Sometimes reaching orgasm is less important than the physical closeness of sex. While women more often seem to be comforted by being held lovingly, men tend to find sexual activity comforting and life-enhancing.

close to your baby—and to your man. You have fulfilled your birthright—that cycle of sexuality that only a woman can know.

Especially for Fathers

Why, you may wonder, should we have a chapter for fathers in a book about breastfeeding? The answer is easy: Because fathers are a vital part of the nursing experience; because it will enrich their lives as well as those of their wives and babies; and because their support and help are needed as much now as they will ever be in their family's life. Fathers are in the unique position of providing a source of strength and balance for their entire family—and to grow through the challenges and opportunities their new role as father affords them.

As a new father, you have embarked upon a new adventure. Like most adventures, it will have its times of exhilaration—and its times of anxiety. Both are normal.

Throughout history most men have hungered to father children and have taken their parenting seriously. Today, however, men in our society seem to have an even deeper involvement in bringing up their children than many did in times past. Our new society-wide appreciation of the father's role in his children's lives acknowledges that his participation in their care is at least as—or even more—important than his traditional responsibility as family breadwinner.

There are some interesting signs of this new appreciation. In public places we see men out alone with their small children. In baby supply stores we see strollers with longer handles

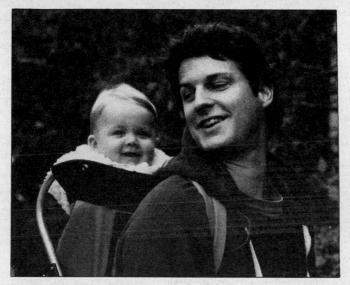

*The father who plays with and cares for
his baby develops a very special attachment
that will enrich both their lives.*

and diaper bags with fewer frills. In television commercials we see fathers diapering and bathing their children. This growth of fathering is bound to enrich the lives of the men doing it, as well as those of their families.

BREASTFEEDING'S BENEFITS FOR YOU, THE FATHER

As the father of a breastfed child, you can appreciate the advantages that nursing confers on your wife and baby. You can also find benefits for yourself, such as the following:

•You don't have to worry about running out of formula at an inopportune time and dashing around trying to find an open store.

•When you go places with the baby, breastfeeding is convenient. There is less to lug—no bottles or cans of formula, no sterilizing equipment. Since the father is usually the one who carries all the paraphernalia required by a new baby, you'll appreciate this lightening of your load when you go on vacation, visiting, or on family errands.

•Breastfeeding puts less of a load on the family budget.

•You can get to know and appreciate a new aspect of your wife's womanliness.

THE FATHER'S IMPORTANCE IN THE FAMILY

A common refrain of many happy breastfeeding mothers is: "I couldn't have done it without my husband's help." While some expectant fathers are afraid they'll feel like a fifth wheel in the family after the baby is born—especially if their wives are nursing—the reality is far different. You are needed. You have a vital role to play in the lives of your wife, your new baby, and your other children. A strong, supportive, helpful husband can often make the difference between breastfeeding success and failure and between family harmony and discord. Let's talk about the different ways you can show this support.

ENCOURAGING YOUR WIFE TO BREASTFEED

Your opinions on breastfeeding are important to your wife, and your encouragement is vital to her success in this endeavor. Before you can encourage your wife to breastfeed your child, however, you have to be convinced of the value of nursing for both mother and baby. You may have some worries about your wife becoming a nursing mother—worries that you can allay by learning more. You'll probably be interested in reading Chapter 1, which discusses the benefits of breastfeeding; Chapter 2, which answers such common concerns as a woman's fear of losing her figure and her fear of being tied down; and Chapter 10, which talks about the sexual relationship between husband and wife.

You can learn a great deal about breastfeeding and other issues related to the arrival of your baby by attending prenatal classes for expectant parents. If you want to be present during your baby's birth, you'll probably have to have some prenatal education before you can obtain permission to stay with your wife during labor and delivery. Even if you're not going to be in the delivery room, you'll still want to learn something about childbirth. Prenatal courses usually discuss breastfeeding and the postpartum period, as well. Another advantage to enrolling in one of these classes is the opportunity to see that you are not alone, that other men share your concerns and confusion.

Sometimes local chapters of such organizations as International Childbirth Education Association, La Leche League, or ASPO/Lamaze hold meetings for fathers, where you can air your questions and receive authoritative answers. Or you may want to take your questions to your doctor or midwife, to your parents, your brother or sister, or perhaps to a friend whose own wife breastfed her children.

BEING YOUR WIFE'S STRONGEST ALLY

Your emotional support and encouragement are even more important to your breastfeeding wife than they would be if she had chosen to bottle-feed. This is because a woman's ability to give milk is so strongly influenced by her emotional state. If your wife is tense after a quarrel or if she senses your resentment toward her nursing the baby, she may react physically as well as emotionally so that her let-down reflex is affected. As a result, the baby goes hungry, the mother gets frantic, and the father is caught in an emotional maelstrom.

The calmer and more relaxed a woman is, the better able she will be to produce and give milk. Even today, when most people accept—or at least give lip service to—the benefits of breastfeeding, your wife may encounter discouragement from relatives, neighbors, her employer, or even her doctor. If *you* wholeheartedly support her desire to breastfeed, she will be better able to handle any outside opposition.

You can support your wife most effectively if you are really convinced that breastfeeding is best for baby and mother. But even if you are not 100 percent convinced, you can appreciate the fact that *she* is and you can show your love by helping her as much as possible. What can you do?

• Let her know that you are happy with her choice.

• Let everyone else know that you stand behind her decision.

• Speak to the doctors—your wife's and the baby's—to tell them you'll help her in any way you can.

• Speak to well-meaning friends and relatives who may be showing their disapproval of breastfeeding or doubting your wife's ability. Be her buffer and protect her against their subtle (and not-so-subtle) disparaging remarks. If you make it plain that your wife is not to be discouraged from nursing, people will probably take their cues from your attitude and will keep any negative opinions to themselves.

• Establish good lines of communication. Sharing thoughts and feelings is the cornerstone of a close relationship, and the timing and manner in which you talk to each other go far in determining the quality of your communication. Husbands and wives need to talk.

As Susan, a mother of three small children, told us, "We didn't do a lot of talking, of sharing our gut feelings until just about the last year. I never said to Bill in the early years, 'I really love you but I need some space now for me.'" Her husband added, "And I never said anything to her about how deprived and left out I was feeling. What we did do was fight. I found a lot to criticize in Susan—the house was a mess; the kids were dirty; I didn't have any clean socks."

Now, after they've begun talking more, Susan says, "Now I realize that it wasn't the socks—it was the sex. Or rather, the lack of it. Now I can let the house go and I don't get those complaints. In fact, he pitches in and does more himself. As hard as it is, we manage to find time and energy for each other—for talking *and* for sex."

Both husband and wife need to feel free to express their worries as well as their joys, their anger as well as their happiness. But because of the great effect the emotions have on the course of breastfeeding, the husband who can defer expressing his more negative feelings at least for the first few weeks after the baby is born will be making a great gift to his baby, as well as his wife. Try to understand why she may be more irritable than usual, why she forgets to do things, why she sometimes seems distracted when you're talking to her.

Remember that your wife is probably busier and more wrapped up in her daily schedule (especially if this is her first baby) than she ever has been before and will ever be again, that the hectic pace of these first few weeks does recede and that she will become more calm and less anxious about her new responsibilities.

So, you see how important your role is in the success of your baby's nursing. All this is not to say that you should stifle all your feelings—only that you try to deal with them in as adult a way as possible and to spare your wife, at least in the first few weeks after your baby's birth, as much emotional upset as possible.

In these especially sensitive early days your wife needs to be cared for lovingly. Even the simplest gestures—like bringing her a glass of juice while she's nursing, bringing home a small gift, offering to go to the store—can go far to make her feel appreciated and to alleviate the common down-in-the-dumps feeling that often follows childbirth.

YOUR BABY'S MOTHER IS STILL YOUR WIFE

One of the most important ways by which you can boost your wife's morale is to keep showing your interest in her as your wife. You are still her man and she is still your woman. You have a relationship that includes more than shared parent-

hood. Your wife needs to know that you still consider her interesting and attractive, that you still value her opinions as much
as ever and that you still share interests besides the baby.

As we point out in Chapter 10, some women find that the
sensuality of lactation makes them more interested in sex with
their husbands, while others find this a time of diminished
sexual interest. Even if your wife is in the latter group and is
not interested in resuming sexual relations as soon as you are
(which is no reflection of her feelings for you), she still needs
to be reassured of your love. This reassurance can take such
physical form as cuddling and kissing even when it does not
include sexual intercourse.

One recent study of 194 couples found that the first sexual experience after childbirth was considered satisfying by
more than two thirds of the new fathers, but by fewer than half
of the mothers. Pain and fatigue are major factors in many new
mothers' more negative experience of sex.

Another major factor in the less satisfying sexual experiences of some women is their feeling about their own attrac-
tiveness. Women who don't like the way they look because
they're heavier than usual, because they have stretch marks,
or because they feel "top-heavy" don't feel like desirable sexual partners. As a result, they may withdraw from sex.

It's clear, then, that there are things that a caring husband can do with regard to all these factors. In the previous
chapter we talked about ways to lessen the discomfort of renewed sexual activity. It's important to realize the problems
this pain causes for some women and to be patient as well as
flexible in your sexual techniques.

You can help your wife feel better about her desirability by
letting her know that you like the way she looks. If you can
accept the fact that she may be heavier than usual throughout
lactation and if you value those curves as symbolic of her fertility and her ability to nurture, you will be helping her to accept
herself, too. One way to show her that you think she's beautiful is to tell her so; another is to take photographs of her, especially while she's nursing the baby. Other ways are to surprise
her with an occasional appearance-related gift, such as a piece
of jewelry or an item of clothing that's becoming as well as
practical.

ROLLING UP
YOUR SLEEVES

While the kind of emotional support we've just been talking about can be enormously helpful to your wife, she's sure to appreciate more practical kinds of help, too. Fortunately, these days there is much less of a sharp distinction between work that's appropriate for either sex. There's no longer any stigma attached to a man's cooking or cleaning, just as there's no stigma attached to a woman's mowing the lawn or putting up storm windows.

Every woman needs a great deal of rest after giving birth. Her body has to recover its strength, even while her sleep is constantly being disturbed. While a run-down nursing mother can produce milk, the effort will take its toll in her own health and in the quality of care she can give to her baby and to the rest of her family. It's essential to see that your wife rests enough.

One of the most important things that you can do as the father of a breastfed baby is to help your wife get the rest she needs at night, especially in the first few months. When your baby awakens during the night, you become the one on call. If your baby is sleeping in a separate bed, you become the one who gets up out of bed, gets the baby, brings him to your wife, and helps her get into a comfortable nursing position. After the feeding, you take the baby back, diaper him, and put him back to bed. By doing this at all nighttime feedings, you'll be performing the vital function of conserving your wife's energy so that she'll be better able to breastfeed—and better able to get through the day. There's no way to overestimate the psychological as well as the practical benefits of this help.

Another way to help your wife conserve her energy is to hire someone to come in to help with the housework for a while if your budget permits. Your investment will pay off in everyone's good spirits and in time both you and your wife can devote to each other. If this is out of the question, pitch in yourself. You can market, cook, vacuum, do laundry, bring home take-out food, and take care of the baby and any other children. As one father told us, "The more I do in the house the better our relationship gets—especially our sex life. My wife isn't as tired, she feels good about herself, and she feels good about me. Besides, it's satisfying to know that I can do things I'd never done before, like whip up a pretty good meal."

YOU CAN BE A COMPLETE FATHER

One common worry among husbands of wives who plan to breastfeed is that there will be no way in which they can help to care for the baby. While this fear is very real to men who want to be actively involved in their babies' lives, it has to bring a smile to the face of any experienced parent. There is so much more to taking care of new infants besides feeding them!

If you want to be close to your baby, you can do so much for her. Just because your wife went through nine months of pregnancy, bore your child, and is now nursing, this does not mean that she is the only person who can care for the baby. You can be just as tender with your baby as any woman might be—with no loss to your masculinity.

What can you do? A lot, as shown in the box on the next page (Some Ways "Breastfeeding" Fathers Can Nurture Their Babies).

You'll want to have some time alone with your baby. This isn't "baby-sitting," which by definition involves taking care of someone else's baby. This is parenting. This is taking care of your own child. This is an activity that knows no gender limitations. You can do your one-on-one parenting between feedings at first, giving your wife a chance to rest or go out while you and your baby enjoy your tête-à-tête. Or you can take the baby out in carrier or carriage. As your wife's milk supply becomes well enough established to miss a feeding (after the first six weeks), you may be giving the baby an occasional bottle, either of breast milk she has expressed and stored, or of formula. For tips on bottle-feeding, see Chapter 9.

At home with your family, and especially with your children, you can let down that protective shell you may wear all day at work. You can free yourself to express those warm, tender expressions of emotion that are yours to give. A man who can freely give and take loving feelings can know completion as a human being.

If you have older children, one of the most meaningful

Some Ways "Breastfeeding" Fathers Can Nurture Their Babies

•Take the baby out of the crib at any time of the day or night to take him to his mother for feedings.

•Change diapers, either before, after, or during the mid-feeding break.

•Walk around with the baby, carrying her in a baby carrier to feel her soft warmth next to you and to let her enjoy your presence.

•Rock or walk him when he's unhappy or soothe him in some other way (as suggested in the box, "Ways to Comfort a Crying Baby" in Chapter 8).

•Enjoy one of the most gratifying activities of parenthood, giving your baby a bath.

•Let your baby fall asleep on your chest, where he's able to hear your heartbeat and feel your warm (and maybe fuzzy) skin.

•Hold and stroke her and show how loving your touch can be.

•Give him a soothing massage.

•Work through some baby exercises with her.

•Sing to him.

•Talk to her. With these last two activities, you'll not only be establishing a relationship—you'll also be helping your baby's language development.

things you can do for them, for your wife, and for yourself is to lavish extra time and attention on them after your wife comes home with the new baby. If *you* as an adult feel pushed to one side, imagine how *they* feel. Plan outings with them when they can have your undivided attention. Offer special treats to show them how important they are to you. The extra time you spend with your older children will mean as much to your wife as to the children themselves, since her mind will be more at ease, knowing that they are happy while she is taking care of the new baby. They'll also provide extra benefits to you as you get to know your children better and reap more of the rewards of parenthood.

As David Stewart, Ph.D., has written in his wise little pamphlet, *Fathering and Career: A Healthy Balance,* "Careers are fickle, but parenthood is forever." As this father points out, while many things in life can wait, the growth of a child is not one of them. "To enjoy a two-year-old," he says, "you must do it when he or she is two."

You can create extra time for your children (which will be meaningful both to them and to you) by waking up earlier or by setting aside time when you come home at night. You can declare a temporary moratorium on overtime, travel, and weekend work. If you consider time with your children a necessity, you'll be able to plan for it in your schedule.

GETTING SUPPORT
FOR YOURSELF

It sounds as if a great deal is being asked of you at this time. You're right. A great deal is. That's why it can be very helpful if you have someone that *you* can turn to for comfort. New fathers need special helpers, too—caregivers who, as we described them in Chapter 4, can offer friendship, reassurance, and both practical and emotional support.

Most new fathers are apt to feel somewhat shut out of the family circle, no matter how their babies are fed. Some men can accept these feelings more easily than others—but virtually *every* new father has them to some degree. You're not abnormal; you're not a selfish brute; you're not immature for experiencing twinges of jealousy and hurt after the birth of your baby. Listen to what one new father has said about what he embarrassedly calls "spousling rivalry": "I feel like a big baby, jealous of my own son. I love the baby, sure, but I miss having a wife who cares about me. She goes on and on about him, which I can understand, but occasionally it would be nice if I got the feeling that she cared how I am."

This is an exceptionally difficult time for both you and

your wife. Your familiar household routines are completely disrupted. You both have to learn how to carry out your roles as parents. You have to take into account the needs and wants of a new person—a completely helpless and very noisy addition to the family. You have new responsibilities toward your wife as she recuperates from the physical demands of pregnancy and childbirth and copes with the hormonal changes accompanying these events. You're likely to feel sexually frustrated. If you have older children, they are apt to be especially needy at this time of family turmoil. Your social life is disrupted, and you may feel you'll never again have the freedom and the fun you and your wife used to have together. In addition, you have new financial strains, especially if your wife had been making a substantial contribution to the family income and is now taking an extended maternity leave. You not only have to cut back to living on one income—you have all the added expenses brought by the baby.

At a time, then, when you have to be more giving to both your wife and your baby, you may feel like being taken care of yourself. Both you and your wife have mixed-up feelings, and each of you needs a lot of moral and practical support.

Many men consider their wives their best friends. This may work at most times in their lives, but when they have an issue they cannot talk to their wives about, they have no one to go to. Often, men are unable to talk to another man about their most deeply felt feelings for fear of showing their vulnerability. Yet as most women have learned, sharing ourselves, including the selves we usually don't show to the outside world, is often a bridge to intimacy with another person, who can then share something of himself.

This may be an ideal time in your life to seek out a man you feel you can trust (if you don't have such a friend already in your life). Some good candidates for such help include your father, brother, or brother-in-law, or clergyman. You'll probably get the best kind of understanding and possibly even practical advice from someone who's already been through this stage in his life, but if you can't find someone like that, you can at least find someone who can turn a sympathetic ear your way and just listen.

The role of fathers in their babies' lives has become a major research interest for many psychologists. They have found that attachments and close ties form between fathers and their children during the first year of the children's lives and that the fathers then go on to exert a strong influence over all aspects of their offspring's development. Anyone who plays a large part in a baby's day-to-day life will have an important influence on that life. After the birth of your new baby, then, you can justifiably feel proud of the major contribution you are making to the lives of your wife and children.

12

Preventing and Treating Possible Problems

You probably won't need most of the information in this chapter or the next. But if you should run into any of the situations covered here, you'll want to know what to do. If your question is not answered here, call your doctor, nurse, midwife, childbirth educator, lactation consultant, or local La Leche League leader.

If you ran into a breastfeeding problem with a previous baby, don't assume that it will occur again. Breastfeeding history does not necessarily repeat itself. Each nursing situation is unique, and now that you're more experienced, breastfeeding is likely to go more smoothly the second time around. Remember, though, that this is a different baby, and that each baby brings his or her own personality, habits, and feeding patterns to the situation, sometimes with problems as a result. Don't blame yourself or your baby if something goes wrong. Just look at the situation as it is and see what you can do about it.

DISAGREEMENT WITH YOUR DOCTOR

Suppose the physician taking care of you or your baby gives you advice that contradicts other information you've received. You may be advised to stop or suspend nursing, you may be told to feed your baby additional formula or solid foods when you want to offer only breast milk, or you may be told to nurse your baby less frequently than you feel is necessary. What do you do?

Relieving Engorgement

- •Express or pump a little bit of milk before feeding, to soften your breasts and make them easier for your baby to grasp.

- •If your breasts are severely engorged, massage them once or twice a day before feeding, starting at the outer edges and going toward the center. A mild cream may make the process easier, but don't get any on the areola, because that would make it harder for you to express any milk.

- •Apply cold or hot packs before a feeding (and before a massage). Both extremes of temperature can help. Some women find more relief in one than the other, and others alternate between the two, generally applying heat before a feeding and cold afterward. Cold can be applied in an ice-pack or a blue freezer-pack wrapped in a thin towel. Heat can be applied in a small hot water bottle wrapped in a towel, a towel soaked in hot water, or in a hot shower. If you use a heating pad, be very careful not to burn your skin.

- •Wear a firm bra for support. Be sure it's not too tight, since this can make you more uncomfortable and also cause other problems.

- •Do *not* use a nipple shield.

First, you want to find out why the doctor is giving you this advice. Is it a consequence of a specific problem that has arisen with either you or your baby? Are you having a problem, perhaps with painful or infected breasts or nipples? Or is your baby jaundiced or not gaining weight at the rate the doctor feels is appropriate? In this chapter we discuss some of these and other problems that may give rise to conflicting advice, and we present the most current remedies for them. Some of these solutions may be at odds with the advice you are receiving. Because each case is unique, however, your own physician is in the best position to evaluate your situation and make recommendations. *If your baby is sick or not thriving or has any special problem, it can be dangerous to disregard medical advice. If you don't have confidence in what your doctor says, find another doctor.* (See Chapter 4.)

But if your baby is healthy and you're well informed, try discussing your differences with your doctor. Some doctors routinely recommend supplementary bottles or early feeding of solids for all their patients, either because of long-established practice or because of their own opinions about desirable lifestyles, which may be different from your own.

One mother approaches such situations this way: "I have found that it's effective to say 'I feel.' If you 'think' or 'insist,' he won't like it. But if you 'feel' you would like to do or not do something, this is a gentle way to open the discussion, because nobody wants to step on your feelings." Another mother who ran into a disagreement with her doctor over breastfeeding her jaundiced baby took in some professional literature supporting her position and said, "I didn't know whether you had seen this recent research recommending that mothers of jaundiced babies continue nursing them. Can you read this and tell me what you think of it?" (The books for professionals listed in the bibliography may be helpful. Also, the medical advisory board of La Leche League International has published materials itself and can refer you to others.)

SORE NIPPLES

Many women experience temporary soreness the first few days after giving birth. If you're not in severe pain and if your discomfort is relieved when your milk comes in and lets down for the baby, you don't need to do anything special. Mild to moderate soreness usually goes away in a few days. But if your nip-

Treating Sore Nipples

•Be sure your baby is properly positioned for nursing, with her body facing yours and her mouth covering all or a good part of your areola, as described in Chapter 7.

•Do not let the baby chew on your nipple.

•Express a little milk manually before putting your baby to the breast to start the milk flowing and to help your let-down operate more quickly.

•Practice a relaxation technique just before nursing. (See Chapter 8.)

•Nurse your baby more frequently, but for shorter periods of time. Your breasts are less likely to overfill and your baby is more likely to suckle gently.

•Limit sucking time to five minutes on the sore side (or on each side, if both nipples are sore). If your baby seems to need more sucking time, give him a pacifier afterwards while continuing to hold him.

•Offer the less sore breast first most of the time. This will give your milk a chance to let down on the sore side, and the baby won't be sucking as hard by the time he gets around to his second course.

•Change your position at each feeding. Lie down, sit up, hold the baby in different positions so that you can equalize the pressure on your breast.

•If a scab forms on your nipple during early nursing, leave it alone.

•If your let-down reflex seems sluggish, ask your doctor to prescribe an oxytocin spray for temporary use.

•To ease pain, apply either ice, crushed and wrapped in a wet washcloth, or gauze squares that have been dampened and put in the freezer, briefly to your nipples, just before a feeding.

•Avoid all irritating substances. Do not use soap, alcohol, tincture of benzoin, or witch hazel on your nipples.

•Do not wipe away milk left on your breast after a nursing. Let it dry there; it may have healing properties.

•Soothe the soreness with a mild over-the-counter ointment such as vitamin A & D, pure lanolin (if you're not allergic to wool), or Massé cream. Wipe it off very gently before the baby nurses. Or apply liquid vitamin E squeezed from capsules, which does not have to be wiped off.

•Keep your nipples dry:

If you wear breast pads to catch leaking milk, change them when they get wet.

If you wear breast shields (milk cups) to bring out inverted nipples, empty them often.

Walk around the house with your nipples uncovered as much as possible.

Undo your bra flaps under your clothing occasionally.

Buy small mesh tea strainers from the five and dime, remove the handle, and insert them in your bra to let air circulate around your nipples while you're dressed.

After nursing or showering, air-dry your nipples with a warm setting on an electric hairdryer.

•Expose your nipples to the light of a 40-watt bulb from a distance of approximately four feet for 4 to 5 minutes four times a day. The gentle warmth is soothing.

•If your nipples are tender after showering, apply a thick coating of lanolin or other thick cream before you take your shower. Wipe it off very gently afterward.

•If the air in your home is very dry (as in an overheated apartment), humidify it by keeping a pan of water on the radiator.

•Occasionally take an aspirin or a glass of beer or wine before a feeding to ease your discomfort.

•Occasionally sore nipples are caused by thrush, a fungus infection in the baby's mouth. Look in her mouth—not right after a nursing, however. If she has milky white spots or a coating on her tongue, gums, or on the insides of her cheeks, call her doctor. While the baby's infection is clear-
(Continued on the next page)

ing up, wash your nipples after every nursing in a solution of one teaspoon of baking soda to a glass of warm water. Dry your nipples gently and apply a mild cream. Wipe it off very gently before nursing.

•Do *not* wear the rubber or soft plastic nipple shields that are sometimes advised to insulate your sore nipples from your baby's sucking. These shields consist of a cone attached to a rubber nipple. The cone fits closely over the breast and the baby sucks from the rubber nipple. They don't provide the stimulation your breasts need to keep making milk, they rarely relieve the soreness, and they cause some babies to develop nipple confusion.

•If, as happens in rare cases, your soreness continues to worsen until the nipple cracks and bleeds and is absolutely too painful to nurse on, take your baby off the affected nipple for 24 to 48 hours. Nurse him on the other breast and, if necessary, give him expressed milk or formula in a bottle. Express or pump your milk every three hours, or every time you would ordinarily be nursing. Gradually resume nursing with short (five-minute) feedings on the sore breast, starting twice a day. Continue to express milk at other feeding times until the breast is healed enough to work up to the full nursing schedule. Apply vitamin E oil and an over-the-counter cream containing one-half-percent cortisone to heal the nipple fissures.

ples look red and chapped or the pain during or after nursing is severe, do something right away. Don't wait until the pain becomes unbearable.

Soreness may set in on the second or third day of nursing, or it may not appear until the second or third week. Or it may not show up at all. While most women experience some discomfort during early nursing, not all do. If you do develop sore nipples, you needn't despair. You can usually heal them quickly and go on to look forward to and enjoy your breastfeeding sessions. See the box on page 244 (Treating Sore Nipples).

Kittie Frantz, R.N., and her colleagues at the University of California Medical Center found that teaching positioning techniques to women with sore nipples almost always reduced or completely eliminated the soreness. So check the way you're holding the baby. Is he in a position so he can get enough of your breast in his mouth without straining? If not, take another look at the pictures and text in Chapter 7 and try repositioning.

Sometimes you may be doing everything right, but your baby may have a sucking problem. Some babies, for example, suck their tongues instead of the breast, or suck their lower lips along with the breast. Others thrust their tongues forward. If your nipple soreness persists, ask someone knowledgeable in lactation to observe you while you're nursing. They may be able to pick up any problems in sucking and give you advice.

ENGORGEMENT (SWOLLEN BREASTS)

The painful swelling of the breasts experienced by some women three to five days after childbirth is caused by a combination of the swelling of the tissues, the increased circulation of blood in the breasts, and the pressure of the newly produced milk. The breasts feel hard, tender, and tight.

The best way to prevent engorgement is to feed your baby as soon after birth as possible and frequently, on demand, from then on. Women whose babies nurse vigorously and often right from the start rarely suffer from engorgement. If you should become engorged, the procedures listed in the box on page 242 (Relieving Engorgement) should help the engorgement to go away in a couple of days.

When it goes away—and it will—be assured that you still have plenty of milk. Once your milk supply is well established, your breasts become soft and stay that way most of the time.

CLOGGED DUCT (PLUGGED DUCT; "CAKED" BREASTS)

In this condition, which can occur anytime during nursing, one or more of the milk ducts are blocked so that the milk

Treating a Clogged Duct

• Be sure your bra (or other clothing, like a sweater) is not so tight that it's pressing on the ducts.

• Breastfeed more often and for a longer period of time, so that your baby can help you empty the breast.

• Change your position with every feeding, so that the pressure of your baby's sucking will hit different places on the breast, exerting pressure on different ducts.

• Express or pump milk from the affected breast after each feeding if the baby has not nursed long and rigorously, to get out as much milk as possible.

• If dried secretions are covering the nipple openings, wash them off very gently after each nursing with a piece of cotton saturated with warm water.

• Offer the sore breast first, so that the baby will empty it better.

• Apply moist heat several times a day (hot water bottle, hot wet towel or wash cloth, or tub bath or shower).

• Get extra rest.

• Do *not* wear a nipple shield, which will make it even harder for the baby to empty the breast.

• Do not sleep on your stomach, putting pressure on the breast.

• Continue to nurse. If you stop suddenly, the breast is likely to get too full, the condition will worsen, and infection may result.

• If the lump remains for more than three days, go to your doctor. While the lump is probably related to breastfeeding, it may not be and should be looked at.

• If you repeatedly suffer from clogged ducts, reevaluate the way you're holding your baby or the way your baby is sucking.

cannot pass through them. You're likely to find a small lump on the breast that's reddened and painful to touch. If not treated, this condition can lead to a breast infection so you should take immediate measures, as suggested in the box on the facing page (Treating a Clogged Duct).

BREAST INFECTION (MASTITIS)

When breast infections occur, they usually show up between two and six weeks after birth, but they may appear earlier or

---

Treating a Breast Infection

- Go to bed immediately and stay there as much as you can.

- Call your doctor right away. You may receive a prescription for an antibiotic or a pain reliever that will be safe to take while you continue to nurse.

- Apply moist heat to the infected breast (hot water bottle or hot wet towel). Do *not* apply an ice-pack.

- Offer the sore breast first at each nursing so that it can be emptied more completely.

- Wear a firm bra for support; be sure it's not too tight.

- Drink plenty of fluids.

- Do not wean suddenly, since this can contribute to an *abscess,* a serious and painful infection that may require surgery and temporary cessation of nursing from the affected breast.

- If you suffer repeatedly from breast infection, check for factors that may be causing it—allowing your breasts to become too full, not alternating them, improper positioning of your baby, inadequate washing of your hands before nursing, using an unclean breast pump, or not getting enough rest. Change what you can and seek help at the first sign of infection.

much later. Symptoms include headache, painful engorgement with the breast hot and tender to the touch, redness, fever, and a generally sick, ache-y, flu-like feeling. Your milk supply may drop. A breast infection may be a complication of a clogged duct or the result of an infection carried from the baby to the mother or picked up elsewhere.

Mothers with breast infections used to be told to stop nursing immediately. We now know that breast infections clear up more quickly and with fewer complications when the mother continues to nurse from the affected breast. There is no danger from the baby's becoming ill from nursing at an infected breast; she probably harbors the same germs in her mouth and nose that may have caused the problem in her mother's breast. Occasionally a baby may not nurse well at an infected breast because the milk tastes salty. If this happens, express or pump from the infected breast and nurse from the unaffected one.

It is important to treat a breast infection right away, as suggested in the box on page 249 (Treating a Breast Infection). With treatment, the fever should drop within 36 to 48 hours, and the soreness and hardness will go away soon afterward.

SUDDEN INCREASE IN BABY'S DEMAND

Your baby may have seemed happy with a nursing schedule that the two of you have worked out, but just as soon as you think you're settled into a routine, he begins to demand more. You wonder what has happened, and you worry that you're losing your milk. This is a fairly common occurrence and nothing to worry about. It can occur for a number of reasons, and is usually easy to resolve. All you have to do in most cases is nurse more frequently for several days. This will build up your milk supply and get your baby over the transition.

One reason why this sometimes happens lies with the baby's growth. Babies grow irregularly. During periods of particularly fast growth, sometimes called "growth spurts," they need more fuel. The most common times for this apparent increase in a baby's need for nourishment are three weeks, six weeks, three months, and six months of age. While you're nursing more frequently, you may also be able to increase your milk supply in other ways. (See Chapter 8.) As your baby approaches six months, you may want to begin feeding solid foods. (See Chapter 14.)

Another reason for what seems like a sudden increase in your baby's appetite may lie with you. Nursing and motherhood may have become so easy and manageable that you forgot to mother yourself. You work more, you go out more, you do more, and you forget about resting enough and eating right. As a result, your milk supply may diminish. This is easy to remedy. Take a look at your life and cut back on outside involvements while you take better care of yourself.

THE BABY WHO GAINS TOO SLOWLY

Occasionally a baby of two or three weeks will have gained practically nothing since birth. Or a baby may have begun to gain and then for no apparent reason hit a plateau. The baby may be crying constantly, obviously hungry all the time. Or he may sleep for several hours at a stretch, nurse well, and seem happy. Either way, it's worrisome. Is the baby sick? Or not getting enough to eat?

Any baby who doesn't gain or seems unhappy much of the time should be examined by a physician. A baby who is sick won't do well at either breast or bottle until his condition is dealt with. If the baby seems well, you should take a look at your own health. Are you feeling well, eating enough, getting enough rest? Are you taking drugs that could interfere with your milk production?

If, as is usually the case, no physical problem is found with either you or your baby, a number of steps can be taken to encourage weight gain and normal growth, as suggested in the boxes on the following pages (Helping the Slow-Gaining Infant, Checking Your Baby's Sucking Technique, and Helping the Older Baby Who Isn't Gaining). The first two discuss problems that show up in the first month of life; the third discusses those that appear after a few months.

Helping the Slow-Gaining Infant

•Look at your breastfeeding patterns:

Is your baby eating every three or four hours, either because she sleeps for several hours at a stretch and doesn't ask to eat, or because you've been encouraging her to go longer between feedings? If so, nurse every hour or two, even if it means waking your baby up every couple of hours during the day.

Has your baby been sleeping more than six hours at night before eight to 12 weeks of age? If so, wake her every four hours at night.

Have you been timing feeding sessions, removing the baby when you think it's time, allowing only 20 or 30 minutes? If so, let sessions run for about an hour.

Has your baby been taking only one breast at a feeding? If so, nurse from both. If she falls asleep after one, burp her and change her and then nurse on the other side. Switch breasts more than once during a feeding. This encourages multiple let-downs and, as a result, more milk.

Is the baby getting milk or water from bottles? If so, your breasts may not be getting enough stimulation, and your baby may be experiencing nipple confusion. Eliminate the water. If the baby needs supplemental formula, feed it

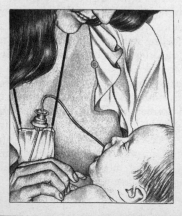

The Lact-Aid Nursing Trainer provides both nourishment and a nursing experience to many babies, including those whose mothers don't seem to have enough milk to foster normal weight gain and those who have not yet mastered efficient sucking techniques.

through a feeding device like the Lact-Aid system, an eye dropper, or a teaspoon.

Remember, though, that neither of the last two methods help the baby learn how to suckle, and the eye dropper approach is potentially hazardous, since there is the risk of dropping more fluid into the baby's mouth than he is able to swallow easily, possibly causing him to aspirate it into the lungs.

Is the baby using a pacifier to fill her sucking needs?

•Suppose you're already doing everything suggested here. If so, the first thing to do is to make *extra* efforts to build up your production of milk. The best way is to nurse more frequently, as often as every hour or two. Other suggestions, as given in Chapter 8, may also help.

•If, after four or five days of this regime, your baby is still not gaining, supplement breastfeeding with formula fed through a feeding tube device such as the Lact-Aid Nursing Trainer.[1] This appliance consists of a collapsible plastic bag with a lid and a long, very thin tube. Formula is poured into the bag, which fits into the mother's nursing bra between her breasts. The tube is placed next to her nipple and held there with surgical tape.

While the Lact-Aid system has been on the market since 1971 and has been proven safe and effective, several other companies have since developed similar devices that use a bottle or other container, with varying degrees of safety and effectiveness.

In this type of system, the baby suckles the breast and the tube simultaneously, receiving milk as soon as she starts to nurse. Because of the way the system delivers fluid to the baby, it provides a type of oral patterning that helps to improve or train the baby's suckling skill and coordination. Meanwhile, the device helps to increase the mother's milk supply, since the baby is stimulating the breasts more effectively. Throughout, the baby is getting the nourishment

---

[1]This system is sold in some local pharmacies and health care supply stores. It is also available by mail order. For information on obtaining it, contact Lact-Aid International, Inc., P.O. Box 1066, Athens, TN 37303, (615)744-9090.

(*Continued on the next page*)

she needs, and both mother and baby are having the experience of nursing at the breast, with all the warmth and intimacy that are such a rewarding part of breastfeeding.

• You need to look at your baby. In some cases, babies fail to gain weight because they have a sucking problem. The quality of a baby's suck is at least as important as the frequency and duration of feeds. Some of the same problems we talked about in connection with sore nipples in the mother can cause poor weight gain in the baby. Fortunately, these problems can often be overcome by changes in positioning or other management of breastfeeding, as suggested in the box on page 256 (Checking Your Baby's Sucking Technique). A doctor, lactation consultant, childbirth educator, or La Leche League leader may be able to help you identify your baby's problem and help you solve it.

THE BABY WHO GAINS TOO FAST

While we used to think it was impossible to overfeed a breastfed baby, an occasional totally breastfed baby seems to be in danger of being overstuffed. This is a baby who is gaining so much weight that he is in the top five percentile of weight for a baby of his length. Most people once thought that a fat baby was a healthy baby, but too much fat is no good. It's not healthy now, and it's possible that it may lead to obesity later in life.

This is not an issue during the first couple of months of life. A very young infant should be fed frequently, with no concern about overfeeding. By the time a baby is three, four, or five months old, however, the mother of an extremely plump baby should ask her doctor whether her baby is getting too fat. This sometimes happens when a mother who has a great deal of milk offers the breast every time her baby opens his mouth, and when the baby is agreeable about taking the breast even when he's not hungry.

Babies cry for all sorts of reasons, many of them entirely unrelated to hunger. Just as it's inappropriate to offer an older

Helping the Older Baby Who Isn't Gaining

Sometimes there's a sudden loss of weight or a failure to gain weight in a baby several months old, who has been doing fine up until now. If this happens, look for the following:

•*Is your baby teething?* If she's drooling a lot and trying to put everything into her mouth, she may be teething and finding nursing uncomfortable. Whenever you see her sucking her fist or fingers, pick her up and nurse her. More frequent short nursings will provide her with the nutrients she needs, while lessening the discomfort. After nursings you can give her ice-soaked teething rings until she seems more comfortable. If she seems extremely uncomfortable, you may ask your doctor for suggestions.

•*Has he become so efficient at nursing* that he zips through his feedings and is ready to stop after five minutes? If so, he may not be getting enough milk. Try burping and switching several times during a session; the new surge of milk after a second let-down may interest him in staying at the breast.

•*Are you doing too much?* Cut back as much as possible on your activities for a while. Rest more, eat and drink more, and take care of yourself, to increase your supply of milk.

•*Is she easily distracted?* Does she break away from the breast to look around and see what's going on around her? Breastfeed in a quiet, dimly lit room.

•*Does he spend many happy hours with a pacifier or sitting in a swing?* Devices like these can be wonderful helpers to a busy mother, but if your baby is showing a weight loss, put them aside for a while. Pacify and amuse your baby more with your breast; when he is once again gaining well, you can reintroduce the other pleasures.

•*Does the baby begin to nurse, then reject the breast?* If so, see the section, Temporary Rejection of the Breast on page 258.

Checking Your
Baby's Sucking Technique

•Pull down his lower lip while he's nursing. Can you see his tongue between his lips and your breast? If not, he may be sucking his tongue. Try putting your index finger on the baby's chin, pressing it down a little. Or put your finger in the baby's mouth, flatten his tongue, and insert your nipple on top. Repeat until he's doing it right. If neither of the techniques works, ask your doctor to look at the tongue; occasionally the membrane tying it to the floor of the mouth is too short and needs to be clipped.

•Does she seem to be sucking her lower lip along with your breast? If so, take her off the breast, start her over again, and pull the lip out after she's attached.

•If your nipple tends to point down, point it straight into the baby's mouth by pressing down on the top of your breast with your thumb.

•If the baby seems to clench his jaws and clamp the end of your nipple, pull down on his jaw with your index finger; when he begins to suck properly, release the pressure.

•Test your baby's sucking technique by the Marmet Suck Assessment: Trim the fingernail on your index finger, wash and rinse your hands, stroke your baby's cheek toward the lips, and when her mouth opens, insert your finger with the nail down. If the baby is sucking correctly, the sides of her tongue will curve around your finger, her tongue will cover her lower gum ridge, you'll feel a sucking motion starting at the tip of her tongue and rolling back with wavelike motion, she'll suck your finger far back into her mouth, your finger pad will touch her soft palate, she won't gag, and she'll suck rhythmically, occasionally resting without breaking suction. If your baby's sucking does not feel like this, she may have a problem with her suck.

•Does the baby arch his back during nursing? If so, he may not get enough of the breast in his mouth. Hold him in the football hold with his feet up behind you so that he can't push against anything.

•Is the baby so excitable that she keeps losing the breast? Try swaddling her.

•Does the baby drink so fast that she swallows a lot of air? Burp her often.

•Some babies become frustrated if the milk does not flow freely. It may help if you express a little bit before you begin to nurse.

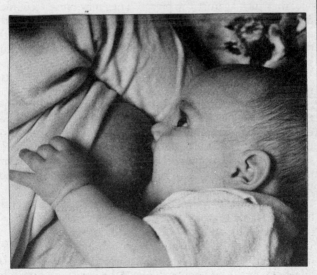

This baby is sucking well, directly facing her mother, taking enough of the breast into her mouth—and obviously enjoying the experience.

child a cookie every time she's unhappy, you don't want to program an infant to satisfy her every want by taking something into her mouth.

If your baby seems too fat, try offering only one breast at each feeding (expressing milk from the other breast if you're uncomfortable). Meanwhile, try to meet the baby's needs in a variety of ways that don't involve feeding him. (See Ways to Comfort a Crying Baby in Chapter 8.)

TEMPORARY REJECTION OF THE BREAST

Sometimes when babies are between four and 10 months of age, they turn against the breast. They may nurse a couple of minutes, then arch their backs and cry. Nothing the mother can do will induce them to go back, and yet it's obvious that they want something. What's wrong? It could be any of a number of things.

If you want to continue nursing, don't start to give bottles now.

If your baby has begun to eat solid foods, increase his portions of these for a few days to tide him over. If he has been eating large amounts of solids, however, this may be causing the problem. He may be too full of food to be interested in nursing. As with so many other childrearing issues, you have to look closely at your own baby and at what is going on in his life.

The box, Why a Baby May Reject the Breast, lists a number of possible reasons for such a development. Express or pump your milk and give it to him in an eye dropper, a teaspoon, or a cup. Meanwhile, keep offering the breast. The most effective time to do this is to pick him up while he's asleep; he won't remember to reject the breast, and once he's back in the routine of nursing, he may decide it's pretty good, after all. If none of them apply to your baby, if after a week she's still refusing the breast, and if she's more than six months old, she may be signaling her readiness to be weaned. While some children want to nurse long after their mothers had thought they would, others surprise and disappoint a mother

Why a Baby May Reject the Breast

•*Is she eating a lot of solid foods?* Cut back on them and nurse more frequently.

•*Has the baby turned against the taste of the milk?* It may have changed because of a cream you're using on your breasts, because of some new food that you're eating, or because you may be pregnant.

•*Is she teething?* If she bit you, she may have been startled by your cry of pain. Also, see the suggestions in Helping the Older Baby Who Isn't Gaining on page 255.

•*Is he wildly hungry?* If he can't seem to wait for the milk to let down, try picking him up about 15 minutes before you would ordinarily feed him, or express a little milk first to give your let-down a chance to work.

•*Does she have a cold?* She may be having trouble breathing through her nose. Try using a vaporizer in the room or ask your doctor whether nose drops would help.

•*Does he have thrush?* This mouth infection, described on page 245, can make nursing painful. If you suspect it, treat it immediately, since the infection can spread to you.

•*Does she have an earache?* If so, it may be painful for her to nurse.

•*Are you under tension or doing too much?* If you're going through a particularly difficult time, your feelings may be coming across to your baby, who in turn becomes too upset to nurse. Make a conscious effort to forget about your cares, at least while you're nursing. You'll enjoy these oases in your life and your baby may be calmer, too.

by wanting to give up the breast earlier than she wants to herself. For suggestions on making the weaning process as comfortable as possible, with the least amount of emotional upset for mother and baby, see Chapter 14.

JAUNDICE

Almost all jaundiced babies can continue to be breastfed. Since there's so much confusion about jaundice, worry about so-called "breast milk jaundice," and misinformation that interferes with the normal course of breastfeeding, let's first define some terms:

Jaundice is a condition in which the skin, the mucous membranes, and the whites of the eyes look yellow because of deposits of *bilirubin*.

Bilirubin is a substance that results from the breakdown of red blood cells. It's normal for these blood cells to be breaking down in our bodies slowly and steadily all the time and to release bilirubin, which is transported through the blood to the liver. In the liver a process takes place that moves the bilirubin along to the intestine and eventually into the bowel, where it leaves the body. Jaundice occurs when the bilirubin accumulates in the body because the red blood cells break down too quickly or because the liver does not process the bilirubin as fast as it should.

Kernicterus is a staining by bilirubin of certain brain tissues. Since it is associated with brain damage, it's fortunate that it is very rare. When it does occur, it is most likely to affect premature babies and babies suffering from pathologic jaundice. Because this condition is so serious, however, it is important to treat jaundice when the bilirubin count approaches high levels.

Types of Jaundice

There are three basic kinds of jaundice:

Physiologic Jaundice. Normal jaundice is common in both bottle-fed and breastfed new babies because their livers are immature; about half of all healthy, full-term newborns become mildly jaundiced. The rate is higher among premature babies. The yellowness of eyes and skin usually appears about the third day after birth. It's harmless and does not need to be treated; it will go away by itself, usually by one week of age in the full-term baby, three or four weeks in the premature. *There is no reason to suspend or stop breastfeeding,* and recent research also shows that there is no benefit to giving supplementary formula or sugar water to jaundiced breastfed babies.

Breast Milk Jaundice. Apparently caused by the presence of a substance in some mothers' milk that either speeds up red cell breakdown or slows down liver function, this type of jaundice appears five to seven days after birth, peaks within three days, and remains for as long as two or three months. *In almost all cases, there is no need to stop or suspend breastfeeding.*

If bilirubin levels are very high, however, some doctors advise temporary interruption of breastfeeding for 12 to 36 hours. This often serves two purposes—diagnosis and treatment. If the count drops, the baby probably has breast milk jaundice. Once the levels have dropped, they may go up again but are not likely to reach the previous high levels. Breast milk jaundice occurs in only about 1 percent of breastfed babies and is not known to lead to any serious difficulties, but because there's no proof that such jaundice cannot become severe enough to cause trouble, it's important to keep a close check on bilirubin levels.

Pathologic Jaundice. This kind of jaundice differs from the first two, both of which are harmless and not symptomatic of any illness. This type results from the too rapid breakdown of red cells, which occurs in some physical conditions, such as an incompatibility in mother-child blood types (Rh factor incompatibility, which can be very severe, is, fortunately, quite rare these days; ABO blood-type incompatibility is milder and commoner), an enzyme deficiency, and certain other disorders. This kind of jaundice may appear on the first day of life and persist for several weeks. Both the condition itself and the jaundice need to be treated. These babies may need breast milk even more than healthy babies do and can and should continue to be breastfed while they are being treated.

Treatment

We now have two excellent ways of treating severely jaundiced babies: *phototherapy*, in which babies are put under high-intensity fluorescent lights or in natural daylight by a window;

and *exchange transfusion*, in which the baby's blood is replaced (most often done in extreme cases of mother-baby blood-type incompatibility). To determine the kind and severity of a baby's jaundice, his blood is tested to measure the bilirubin levels. If they are high, treatment—usually phototherapy—is called for. At one time jaundiced babies were given water to flush out their red blood cells, but we now know that that is unnecessary.

You can continue to breastfeed during the testing and treatment periods. If your doctor recommends phototherapy for your baby, find out how this is managed in your hospital. The baby does not need to be under the lights all the time, so your breastfeeding schedule should not be disrupted. You can continue to nurse on demand, except for the periods when your baby is under the lights. If you have rooming-in, you may be able to have the lights brought into your room. The lights tend to make babies lethargic, so you may have to wake your baby every two hours to nurse.

If your jaundiced baby is healthy in every other respect, you should be able to take her home with you at the normal time of discharge, even though you may have to bring her into the hospital for blood tests to monitor the bilirubin levels. If your doctor feels the baby should still be receiving phototherapy, you can do this at home, either with new fluorescent lights tubes or in ordinary daylight (not direct sunlight; babies' skin burns easily) until the levels drop.

In almost all cases you can continue to nurse your jaundiced baby. Even if your baby needs to remain in the hospital, you may be able to go there to nurse him for some feedings and to leave your expressed milk for him for others. The only time your doctor may want you to interrupt giving your milk to your baby would be to diagnose whether his jaundice is due to breast milk or to some other cause, or in the presence of very high bilirubin levels caused by breast milk jaundice. If such an interruption is called for, you should pump or express your milk to maintain your milk supply. You can freeze this milk for later use, since restriction of breast milk would be very short-lived. (See the Appendix for suggestions on expressing and storing breast milk.)

13

Special Situations

While the situations described in this chapter are not encountered by most women, they're common enough to rate some mention. If you need more information about any of these topics, you may want to call your doctor, nurse, midwife, childbirth educator, lactation consultant, or local La Leche League leader. Or you may find answers to your questions in one of the more specialized books listed in the bibliography.

BREASTFEEDING THE PREMATURE INFANT

If your baby is born early, you should still be able to breastfeed her, even though you may have to wait awhile before you can actually put her to your breast. Procedures for feeding a premature baby vary, depending on the baby's size, strength, and special needs. If she is very tiny, she may not be able to suck at all; she may have to be fed by *gavage* (a tube that goes from the nose into the stomach) for several weeks until she becomes strong enough to nurse, first from a bottle and then, once she's taking a bottle at every feeding, from the breast. Or your baby may be technically classified as premature, but be well-formed and strong and lack only a few ounces to be considered nor-

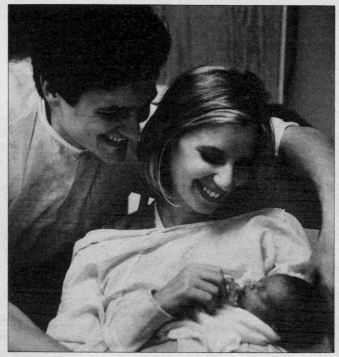

*Frequent visits to the premature nursery help
parents and baby to become a loving
family even before the baby can come home.*

mal. In this case, you can probably start to nurse immediately.

Neonatologists disagree on the best milk for the very small premature baby. This is largely because they don't know how to set a standard for normal growth: Should this baby grow at the same rate that he would if he were still in the uterus? Or at the rate that a full-term baby would? Small preemies grow the fastest when fed special, high-protein formulas. This, however, taxes their bodies' capacities to dispose of the end products of the high-protein intakes, with some danger to their brain development. Furthermore, this route deprives them of the protective factors in breast milk. Some current research efforts are focusing on fortifying fresh human milk with protein, calcium, and sodium in amounts that would meet intrauterine needs.

For the time being, however, whether your baby will be fed your own breast milk or a special high-protein formula depends, again, on your baby's size and strength, and also on your doctor's and your hospital medical staff's philosophy. Because of recent research findings, more physicians now favor feeding premature babies their own mothers' milk. This is because we now know that the milk of women who bear premature babies differs in several ways from the milk produced by women who deliver at term. Thus, your milk is better for your baby than the milk he could get from a milk bank, which pools the milk from different women (usually mothers of older full-term babies, who are producing more than their own babies need).

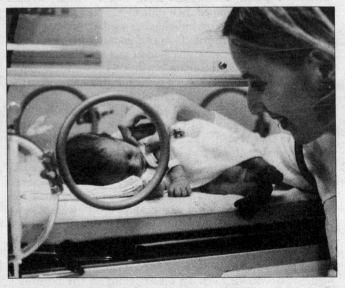

Even a premature baby in an isolette can often be fed his mother's milk, which is specially suited for his growth needs.

The milk of a mother of a premature baby is specially suited for her own tiny infant. It's easier to digest and better constituted for developing the preterm baby's brain and nervous system than is the milk of a mother of a full-term baby. Milk from mothers of preemies has higher levels of nitrogen, protein, lactose, sodium, and chloride than full-term milk. It also has a high level of *lipase,* an enzyme that aids in fat absorption, and studies have shown that preemies who receive a combination of low-birthweight formula and their own mothers' fresh, unheated milk absorb fat better than those fed heat-sterilized human milk (the kind offered from pooled donors' milk) or formula alone. Since these babies need to put on fat, this is an important advantage.

So whether your baby gets your own breast milk right from the beginning or not until he has achieved a certain size and strength, you *will* be able to breastfeed him. Remember that the prematurity is a temporary condition, but that the breastfeeding can continue for many months. Many women have expressed or pumped their milk for the first several weeks of their babies' lives. This milk has been fed to the baby either by tube or bottle, assuring them of a good start in life. After the baby has become stronger, mother and baby have gone on to forge a fulfilling, satisfying nursing relationship. As one mother said, "Breastfeeding a premature baby means a few weeks of uncertainty and inconvenience, followed by many months of blissful happiness, contentment, and satisfaction."

This route is eminently do-able—but it does take time, effort, patience, persistence, and most of all, determination. It's much easier if you can marshal sources of support from your family, your friends, hospital personnel, and breastfeeding consultants. Many women are grateful that they persisted through the early difficult times until they were able to establish a normal breastfeeding relationship. Other women, who found it too difficult to maintain the kind of schedule required early on and switched to formula, feel that the breast milk their babies received in their first days or weeks of life gave them a better start than they would have had without it. Some women who decided against breastfeeding at the beginning changed their minds later and were able to relactate, a process described later in this chapter.

Parents of premature babies often experience a welter of

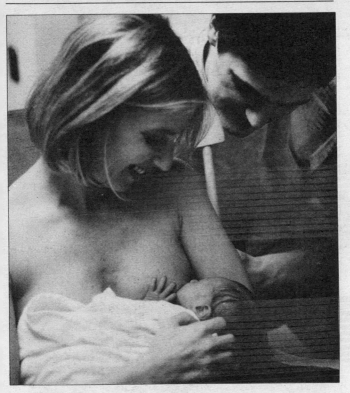

Breastfeeding in the premature nursery is easier when there's a comfortable chair for mother and a welcoming attitude for father.

upsetting emotions. You're likely to be disappointed, worried, confused, and exhausted until the day you feel your baby is out of the woods and will survive, healthy and happy. All these feelings are normal. It will be easier for you to get through these early, difficult times if you get as much support as you can, take as good care of yourself as you can, remind yourself that medicine can do more today for premature babies than ever before, and look forward to the day when your baby will have made up for his hurry to come into this world.

Many women find that offering their milk to their babies

Nursing Your
Premature Baby

LINK UP WITH A SUPPORT SYSTEM

•As soon as possible, contact your childbirth educator, an organization for parents of babies with special needs,[1] a local La Leche League leader, or another mother who has breastfed a premature baby. Your doctor or nurse may be able to put you in touch with someone.

•Let your family and friends know that you plan to breast-

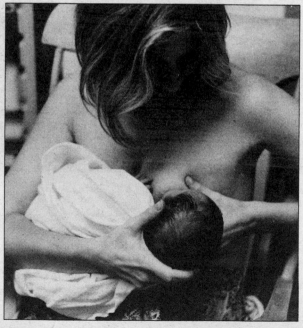

This mother is helping her premature baby by the way she's holding him and her breast. She's keeping his head steady and supporting and guiding her breast.

feed your baby because you believe that breast milk is the best thing for a preemie. Surround yourself with people who will help and encourage you; stay away from those who question and doubt.

BEFORE YOUR BABY IS ABLE TO NURSE

•Ask hospital personnel what arrangements can be made to feed your baby your own expressed milk—where and how you should bring it, how it will be stored, both at home and in the hospital, and so forth.

•Borrow or rent an electric breast pump, which greatly simplifies the task of expressing milk (see the Appendix).

•Begin to express or pump milk on the day after delivery.

•Try to express or pump every two and a half to three hours. This will build up your production now and in the future.

•If the hospital is feeding your baby a special high-calorie formula and you're expressing only to maintain your milk supply until he will be able to nurse, it will be enough to pump every four hours. You can freeze this milk for use later on (see the Appendix).

•Find out your best way to manage nighttime expression. Some women produce more milk if they sleep longer at night, while others do better if they wake up once or twice during the night to express.

•Don't be discouraged if you're not producing as much milk as you would like. Once your baby begins to nurse, you'll have more. Meanwhile, whatever you're giving him contains precious antibodies, nutrients, and enzymes.

•Don't be alarmed about ups and downs in your milk supply. Every woman has them; women who express their milk are more aware of the variations.

---

[1]Parent Care (University of Utah, Health Science Center 2A210, Salt Lake City, UT 84132) offers information, referrals, and other services to parents of infants who need special care at birth.

(Continued on the following pages)

•Expect a drop in milk supply if you're still pumping after several weeks (because no pump stimulates the nipples the way a baby does.) Your production will rise again once your baby begins to nurse.

•If your baby is being fed by bottle, ask whether contoured nipples (like the Nuk or the Kip) can be used, since they force the baby to open her mouth wider and are more like the breast nipple.

•Your menses may return while you're pumping your breasts, since there may not be enough stimulation to suppress menstruation and ovulation. Once your baby is nursing regularly, your menses may stop again, not to resume for several months. Either way, it is possible to get pregnant at this time (see Chapter 10).

BREASTFEEDING IN THE HOSPITAL

•If your hospital will not let your baby leave the nursery to breastfeed, ask whether there's a spot in there where you can nurse.

•Choose a time when your baby is awake and alert, but is not yet crying from hunger.

•Ask for a comfortable armchair.

•Get in a comfortable position. Put one or two pillows on your lap to raise the baby to breast height.

•Make a special effort to relax your face, neck, shoulders, and arms. Take a few slow, deep breaths before you begin.

•If the nursery nurse is supportive of breastfeeding, ask her to help you position your baby and to sit with you the first few times.

•Experiment with different positions. The football hold is good for tiny babies. Another good position involves extending your arm (the one opposite the breast you're nursing) under the baby's back and neck and holding his head steady with your hand. Then move him to a sitting or half-sitting position.

•Make your nipple as easy as possible to grasp, pinching it

to make it longer. (If necessary, wear milk cups before the feeding.)

•Use your thumb and forefinger to keep the breast away from the baby's nose and to support the breast.

•If you're not sure whether the baby can suck and swallow well enough, offer a breast from which milk has just been expressed so that not too much will pour into the baby's mouth.

•Express a few drops of milk into the baby's mouth to whet her appetite.

•Consider the first few nursings "practice feeds." If the baby does no more than lick the nipple a few times, count this as a good beginning. Many babies take a while to learn how to suck; premature babies often need extra learning time.

•If your baby falls asleep at the breast, try burping and switching. Or offer the other breast after an hour or two.

•Expect the first few feedings to be short, possibly two or three minutes, since a small baby tires easily.

•If you have difficulty getting started, ask for privacy. You may do better when you and your baby are alone.

•Push to stay with your baby as much as possible. If your baby has to stay much longer than you do, try to obtain permission to stay overnight for a few nights just before his discharge. This will help you learn his rhythms and begin to establish breastfeeding while you still have the nurses to help you. If there are no regular facilities, ask whether you can sleep on a portable cot or a reclining chair in a room not used in the evening and night, such as an office or a conference or treatment room.

•A growing number of hospitals are letting parents stay with their young children, either before initial discharge or upon a child's later admission to the hospital. If this is impossible, you may still be able to visit several times a day and nurse your baby at those times, and pump or express your milk at the times of any missed feedings.

(Continued on the next page)

•If supplements are required, see whether gavage can be used instead of bottles, to minimize nipple confusion.

WHEN YOUR BABY COMES HOME

•Keep your rental breast pump for at least a week or two after the homecoming. If your baby has too weak a suck to give your breasts enough stimulation, pumping after feedings will help you build production. It will also give you additional milk to supplement nursings if you need to.

•Nurse frequently—every one and a half to two hours for the first day or two, then every two to three hours (eight to 10 times a day).

•If you need to supplement, use the Lact-Aid (see Chapter 12), a teaspoon, or an eye-dropper. Or offer one and a half to two ounces of milk in a bottle (with a contoured nipple) in a separate feeding. (Giving a bottle immediately after a nursing conditions the baby to wait for the bottle.) Gradually eliminate these supplementary bottles.

•Take good care of yourself: Sleep when the baby does; get as much help as possible with the housework; take as long a leave from work as you can. Try not to do anything but feed your baby until he is stronger and the breastfeeding is well established (which may not be until the baby's actual due date).

makes them feel like better mothers, knowing they're providing a special resource that no one else can give. If you do decide to breastfeed your premature infant, you don't need to make a long-term commitment. Even if your baby gets breast milk for only a week or two, she will benefit, and you'll know that you contributed something very special to this small life. All the time, keep your ultimate goal in mind—mothering a healthy, happy baby, and enjoying the relationship.

If you decide to breastfeed, tell your baby's doctor right away and ask for help in doing it. She or he is the one who makes arrangements for your baby to receive your expressed milk or for you to come in to nurse your baby. The two of you will be in close daily touch about the baby's progress. You'll find it easier to nurse your premature baby if you follow the guidelines given in the box on page 268 (Nursing Your Premature Baby).

SEPARATION OF MOTHER AND BABY

Occasionally emergencies come up that separate a breastfeeding mother and her baby for a period of days or weeks. If you want to continue nursing past this separation, it can be done. If you want to wean your baby before the separation, plan ahead, if possible, so that you can do it gradually. If you do wean, you may be able to relactate later, as described at the end of this chapter.

If the separation is caused by your baby's hospitalization, try to obtain permission to stay with him and to nurse him in the hospital. If it's impossible for you to nurse your baby, see whether you can rent an electric pump so that you can express your milk and resume breastfeeding when your baby returns home.

If *you* must be hospitalized, and if your condition permits, you may be able to have your baby come to stay with or visit you in the hospital. If this is impossible, ask your doctor to leave orders and make arrangements so that you can pump your breasts regularly during your hospital stay. Meanwhile, you may be able to find another nursing mother who can feed your baby while you're away. (Your pediatrician or local La Leche League leader may know someone.) If not, your baby can be fed by bottle, either with your own breast milk that you have previously expressed and frozen or with formula.

ILLNESS OF THE MOTHER

If you have some condition that raises questions about the ability or advisability of your nursing your baby, ask your doctor and your baby's doctor. You might also check with La Leche League International (address on page 56), which is apt to have the most current information on medical issues. As of this writing, recommendations can be made for the following conditions:

Herpes

Two kinds of herpes virus that can be passed from mother to baby either during vaginal delivery or through breast milk are cytomegalovirus (CMV) and herpes simplex virus (HSV). CMV is the commoner, less harmful kind, which does not pose a problem to the typical full-term newborn. HSV, however, poses more risks. The herpes simplex virus can cause cold sores or fever blisters on the lips, face, and mouth, or the same type of sore in the genital area. It can be spread through sexual relations with someone who has an active infection, or from an infected person's mouth to her own genitals or eyes if she touches the sores with her fingers.

While much research still needs to be done on this condition, at this time the following guidelines seem useful:

•If you do not have herpes, don't have sexual relations with anyone in an active stage of the disease, especially while you're pregnant or breastfeeding.

•If you have already contracted herpes, get periodic exams and cultures before delivery. If you have an active outbreak, or are in the stage just before sores are apt to break out, tell your doctor. It may be safest for you to have a cesarean birth.

•If you're having an outbreak right after birth, be careful that the baby does not come into contact with any sores or with clothing that has been worn over them. Wash your hands after you go to the toilet and before you nurse, and when you hold your baby drape a clean towel or robe over your lap.

•If you have sores on your breast, postpone nursing until they are fully healed. Until then, express or pump your milk (to build up your supply) and throw it away, and feed your baby by bottle in the meantime.

•If you have an active outbreak when your baby is older, continue to nurse, keeping your baby away from any sores.

Hepatitis B

This virus, which affects about 150,000 Americans each year, appears in breast milk and may be transmitted to a nursing baby. The chances are that the baby of a mother who has hepatitis B will have already been exposed to the virus during pregnancy or delivery. Today many obstetricians test for hepatitis B, especially in populations at high risk for this virus. When a pregnant woman tests positive for the hepatitis B antigen, her baby can receive both gamma globulin and the first of three doses of a new hepatitis B vaccine immediately after birth to protect the baby from contracting the condition. If this kind of preventive care is available, it is probably safe for a mother with hepatitis B to nurse her baby. Since each case is different, however, if you suspect or know that you have been exposed to hepatitis B, you should discuss your situation with your baby's doctor.

Breast Cancer

A number of research studies have tried to find a correlation between breast cancer and breastfeeding. While the findings are somewhat contradictory, the best available evidence seems to be the following:

•Breastfeeding has no relation to the possibility that a woman will develop breast cancer after menopause. Some evidence, however, has been found to suggest that women who breastfeed are less likely to develop breast cancer before menopause. This may mean that breastfeeding *may* help to protect them, or that precancerous conditions may interfere with breastfeeding. So far, we don't know which.

•There is no evidence that women transmit any cancer-causing factors to their babies through breast milk.

•If a malignant tumor is found in a pregnant or lactating woman, its surgical removal should be carried out immediately. Waiting can be dangerous for the mother.

•As of this writing, there is no conclusive evidence as to the safety or danger of the mother's breastfeeding from one breast only after the surgical removal of the other breast because of a diagnosis of breast cancer. The number of women who would have this concern is very small, since most mastectomies are performed on women past their childbearing years. In the absence of large-scale statistical studies, most advice on this topic is based on opinion rather than facts.

Some physicians advise women who have had breast cancer not to get pregnant and not to breastfeed, because both these activities stimulate hormones that could activate cancer cells. Several large studies have shown, however, that pregnancy after diagnosis of breast cancer does not increase the chance of cancer's recurrence and does not affect the woman's survival rate. Waiting to conceive for three to five years after treatment for breast cancer is recommended, since this is the time span when the risk of recurrence is greatest. Some authorities believe that if a woman in this situation does become pregnant, she can go ahead and breastfeed. At the moment, there's no evidence to indicate that this would be harmful to mother or baby.

•While the evidence is inconclusive, research performed to date suggests that if there is any relationship at all between breastfeeding and breast cancer, it is in the direction of lactation's offering some benefit to the mother.

BREAST SURGERY

If you had surgery to make your breasts either larger or smaller, you may be able to breastfeed, depending on the kind of procedures that were followed. In recent years more plastic surgeons have made efforts not to sever or block the milk ducts. For specific information, ask the doctor who performed your surgery, and even if you're doubtful, go ahead and try to breastfeed. It can't hurt the baby. Lactation may well proceed normally, and if it doesn't you can always switch to the bottle.

Breast Augmentation

If you had silicone implants to make your breasts larger and if the implants do not come into contact with mammary tissue, you can probably breastfeed. The procedures in most common use today do not damage the milk ducts. Even if some of the silicone leaks into the milk, this should not be harmful, since the substance is very similar to the main ingredient in a medication often given to babies who are troubled by excess stomach gas. There is no evidence that any babies have been harmed by such leakage.

Breast Reduction

If you had surgery to make your breasts smaller and if the nipple/areola complex is still attached to the breast tissue beneath it, you can probably breastfeed. While the newer procedures are more likely to permit breastfeeding than previous techniques did, there's still a significant chance that breast reduction may interfere with your ability to nurse. If you're considering this surgery, it's probably better to wait until after your childbearing years if you want to be sure you can nurse your babies.

TWINS AND MORE

If you have twins, you don't have to wonder if you should offer one or both breasts at a feeding; you have been designed with perfect efficiency for just this possibility. Furthermore, since breastfeeding operates on a supply-and-demand principle, your breasts should produce ample supplies of milk for both babies. Since babies born in multiples are likely to be small, they derive special benefits from breast milk.

You'll probably find it easiest to nurse both babies simultaneously for most feedings, even though you'll want to nurse them individually occasionally, so that each one will have a chance from time to time to enjoy your undivided attention. Then there will be times when one twin is desperately hungry—and the other sound asleep. As a general rule, you can try letting the hungrier twin set the pattern. When you're about to feed him, wake his twin at the same time. This works best, of course, if both babies are about the same size.

Try to alternate breasts and babies, so that the same twin doesn't always drink at the same fount. But if each baby de-

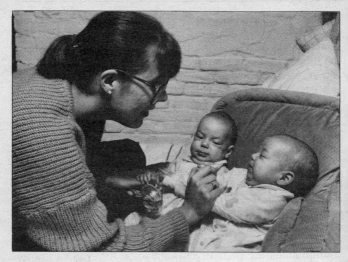

When both twins are about the same size,
like these, they can be on similar schedules,
leaving more time free just for play.

velops a preference for her own side, don't worry about it. If one eats more than the other, you may be a little bit lopsided as long as you're nursing, but you'll return to your former symmetry when they're weaned.

You'll have to work out your own individual schedule. Some mothers nurse twins or even triplets totally, never giving any of the babies a bottle. Others alternate bottles of formula right from the start, rotating between breast and formula (Baby A gets the breast at one feeding, Baby B the bottle; they switch at the next feeding). You need to weigh the benefits of breast milk for your babies with the demands on your own energy and time, and do what's best.

You can get help from The National Organization of Mothers of Twins Club, 5402 Amberwood Lane, Rockville, MD 20853; (301)460-9108. Through this group you can learn of local chapters that will put you in touch with other mothers of multiples. A good source of books about parenting multiples is the Center for Study of Multiple Birth, Suite 463–5, 333 E. Superior St., Chicago, IL 60611; (312)266-9093.

NURSING THROUGH A PREGNANCY AND TANDEM NURSING AFTERWARD

If you become pregnant while you're nursing, your baby may decide to wean, either because your milk tastes different or because there's less of it. Or you may take the initiative in weaning your nursling because of breast or nipple pain, because you're tired, or because you're uncomfortable with the idea. Around the world, a new pregnancy is among the commonest reasons for weaning. Some women do, however, continue to breastfeed throughout pregnancy, and continue to nurse both the older child and the infant afterward. This latter practice is known as "tandem" nursing.

Why do mothers do this? They cite the continued needs

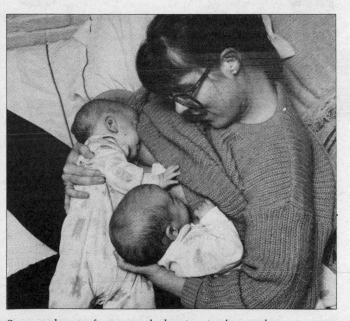

Some mothers prefer to nurse both twins simultaneously; others find it easier and more satisfying to feed one at a time.

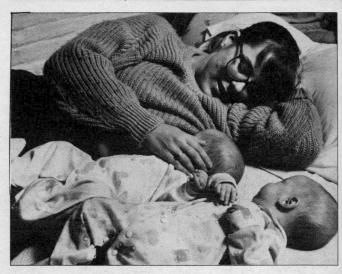

*Sometimes one twin is hungrier than the other;
if either one develops a preference for one breast,
this may result in temporary lopsidedness, but
the mother eventually resumes her symmetry.*

of the older child, whose emotional need for nursing is heightened rather than lessened by the arrival of the new baby, and the mothers themselves sometimes find that they're not ready to sever the nursing tie. Still, tandem nursing mothers often have ambivalent feelings, sometimes resenting the older child, questioning the wisdom of what they're doing, and dealing with the doubled demands on their body.

Some of the challenges facing such a mother include the need for extra nutrition and extra rest to meet the increased demands on her body, first of the pregnancy and then of the nursing infant. While she's pregnant, she needs to find comfortable nursing positions and maternity clothes compatible with nursing. After the new baby is born, she needs to ensure that the new baby gets his rightful share of the colostrum and the milk and she needs to be aware of the danger of crossinfection between both children. This is not a decision to be undertaken lightly, and it is certainly not for everyone. There's

Nursing Two Babies
at the Same Time

When breastfeeding two babies simultaneously, position is everything. Ask someone to help you get the babies set for the first few times, as in the following positions. Experiment until you and the babies are comfortable. Find a comfortable armchair and a couple of pillows. Then try one of these:

• Half-recline and lay each baby on the side or stomach lengthwise along your body.

• Sit up and tuck each baby under an arm, heads resting on firm pillows on your lap and feet by your back (the football hold).

• Hold Baby A on your lap and criss-cross Baby B across Baby A's body.

• Hold Baby A on your lap and tuck Baby B under your arm.

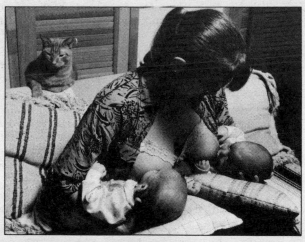

Most mothers of twins experiment till they find the nursing position they—and the babies—like best.

Succeeding at Induced Lactation or Relactation

- Ask yourself *why* you want to do this. If you'll be happy with the experience of nurturing your baby *at* the breast, and not necessarily nourishing him *from* the breast, you're likely to have a more positive experience than if you have your heart set on providing a set amount of milk, or all of your baby's nutritional needs.

- Be prepared for a stressful first few weeks, during which time your baby may resist suckling at the breast, your milk may be slow in coming in, and you'll be nursing almost constantly around the clock and supplementing your baby's diet with formula.

- Find a support system, consisting of people who'll encourage and help you through the difficult days. These people can consist of your husband, doctor, lactation consultant, and, most important, another woman who has done what you want to do, either relactated or nursed an adopted baby.

- You'll find it easiest to relactate if your baby is between four and seven weeks of age, and hardest if she is more than three months old.

- Expect initial resistance from your baby, who is used to getting milk some other way. It may take a week or longer for him to nurse well, but after that he is very likely to become an avid nurser. Don't give up too soon.

- Nipple stimulation is the most important mechanism for bringing in your milk. The best kind of stimulation is your baby's suckling. Other additional techniques include breast massage, nipple rolling, and hand expression or breast pumps. (Milk thus expressed can be fed through the Lact-Aid.)

- Nurse your baby frequently, on demand. In one study, most of the babies nursed eight times a day, at intervals of two to three hours, with two night feedings. (This is an average; some babies need to nurse more often than this at the beginning.) The average duration of each feeding was about 20 to 25 minutes.

•The most popular form of supplementing the baby's diet is the use of a device like the Lact-Aid system (see Chapter 12). This ensures your baby of adequate nutrition while providing stimulation to your nipples. Many women who considered their experience highly successful continued to use the Lact-Aid throughout the course of breast-feeding.

•Other methods of supplementing your baby's milk supply include a nursing bottle, a combination of the Lact-Aid and a bottle, a spoon, syringe, or eye-dropper.

TECHNIQUES THAT ARE HELPFUL INCLUDE:

•increasing your fluid intake and the amount of protein in your diet;

•using an oxytocin nasal spray before putting your baby to the breast, for the first couple of weeks or so;

•asking your doctor to prescribe some other drug, like chlorpromazine or theophylline for the first week or so;

•stroking your baby while she's nursing may help you to relax and let down your milk.

TECHNIQUES THAT ARE NOT HELPFUL INCLUDE:

•keeping the baby hungry to try to encourage him to nurse;

•using nipple shields;

•for adoptive mothers, trying to stimulate the breasts with the nursing infants of friends (the babies usually refuse to suck at a breast that's not producing milk).

no evidence, however, that the practice is harmful to the new baby if his needs are kept paramount.

RELACTATION AND NURSING AN ADOPTED BABY

Sometimes a woman decides or is advised not to breastfeed her newborn infant, or she begins to nurse and then stops for one reason or another. Then, as soon as one week or as late as several months later, she wants to nurse, either because her baby has grown stronger and is now able to nurse, because he has a digestive or allergic problem, or for some other reason. In such a case, it is often possible to initiate breastfeeding. This process is known as *relactation*. In other cases, women who have adopted babies have been able to lactate, even if they have never been pregnant or have not been pregnant for years. This process is called *induced lactation*.

Neither of these processes is easy; both call for a great deal of time, effort, and dedication. Many women who have made the effort, however, have been happy with their decision, especially if they look at it in terms of the enhancement of the mother-baby relationship, rather than any quantifiable measures like the amount of milk they produce, the ability to provide *all* their baby's milk, or the length of time they nurse their babies. Based on several studies of such women, the guidelines given in the box on page 282 (Succeeding at Induced Lactation or Relactation) should help to achieve a happy nursing relationship.

14

Weaning Your Child

Weaning is the process by which your baby stops depending on your milk for nourishment. Thus, your baby is fully weaned when she no longer nurses at the breast, but gets *all* her food from other sources. Before that time, however, your baby will be getting some foods and nutritional elements besides breast milk. Let's take a look at some of these other sources.

OTHER ELEMENTS OF YOUR BABY'S DIET

Vitamin Drops

Most of your baby's vitamins will come through your milk and later through the food he eats, rather than from vitamin drops or pills. There are some elements, though, that cannot always be obtained in the diet. Considerable controversy exists in the medical community about the extent of vitamin supplementation needed by breastfed babies. It's our judgment that the recommendations, which are summarized in the box on page 287 (Recommended Vitamin and Mineral Supplementation), are wise to follow.

During the first six months of life, your totally breastfed

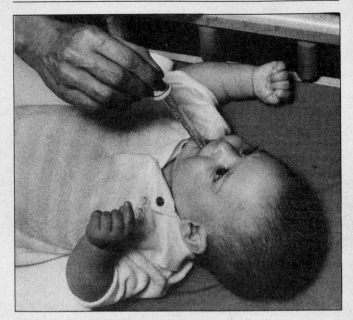

Most babies lick their lips over the taste of vitamins, which is often the first non-breast-milk addition to their diet.

baby may receive enough vitamins from your milk if your own intake is high enough. If, however, you're not sure whether you're eating enough fruits and vegetables, ask your doctor whether your baby should receive a multiple vitamin preparation that includes vitamins A and C.

Vitamin D is especially important since it helps your baby absorb calcium and phosphorus, essential elements for bone and tooth growth and development. Both you and your baby need this vitamin, which appears in only tiny amounts in any food, including breast milk. Vitamin D is called the "sunshine" vitamin, since it's manufactured by our bodies when we spend a great deal of time outdoors and expose our bodies to sunlight.

Many mothers and children can get enough vitamin D from sunshine, but some do not. Dark-skinned people do not absorb as much from the sun because of their deeper pigmentation; high levels of air pollution block transmission of vitamin D to residents of some urban areas; and mothers and babies who do not go out of doors often enough, or who are bundled up by layers of clothing when they do, lessen their exposure to the sun, and thus to vitamin D.

People in the above categories may need extra vitamin D. If you're not in any of these categories, you probably don't need it, but again it can't hurt to be on the safe side. The drops are harmless, inexpensive, and convenient. You should be sure of getting adequate vitamin D throughout pregnancy and lactation, and if your baby's doctor recommends it for her, she can begin taking it from the seventh to tenth day of life.

If your community's water supply contains less than 0.3 ppm (parts per million) of *fluoride*, your baby will benefit from

Recommended Vitamin and Mineral Supplementation

BREASTFED CHILD	MULTIVITAMIN/ MULTIMINERAL	VITAMINS A C D	MINERALS	
			IRON[1]	FLUORIDE[2]
Full-Term Infant	No	Sometimes	No	Yes
Premature Infant	Yes	Yes	Yes	Yes
Healthy Baby (Over 6 Months)[3]	No	Sometimes	Yes	Yes
High-Risk Baby (Over 6 Months)[3]	Yes	Sometimes	Yes	Yes
Healthy Child (Over 2 Years)[3]	No	No	No	Yes
High-Risk Child (Over 2 Years)[3]	Yes	No	No	Yes

[1] Iron-fortified cereal is the preferred form of supplementation.

[2] If child drinks water with a fluoride content over .3 parts per million, additional supplement is not needed.

[3] These recommendations apply if the child is eating a well-balanced diet of solid foods at this time.

a fluoride supplement. If he doesn't drink much water, a fluoride supplement is beneficial even if your water contains a higher level than this. You can find out the level of fluoride in your water by calling your local health department. There's some question whether the fluoride in the water that a nursing mother drinks passes through the milk in sufficient amounts to help her baby develop decay-resistant teeth, and since research has shown that children who get extra fluoride (either in the water or in drops) develop fewer cavities, you'll want your children to have this advantage. The fluoride may be included in your baby's vitamin D drops and may be begun soon after birth, or not until six months of age.

While breast milk contains little *iron*, it is present in a very easily absorbable form. This iron, plus the stores your baby is born with, will see him through his first four to six months. After this time, he'll need some extra iron. The best way to get this is through an iron-fortified baby cereal. If your baby is under six months when you first offer cereal, make it with expressed breast milk, water, or formula; after this time you can use homogenized milk.

Other Milk

If you offer anything other than breast milk in the first few months of life, you should be giving your baby a specially constituted infant formula. This will probably have a basis of cow's milk, with some added ingredients. If your baby has special needs, your doctor may recommend a modified-protein formula or one with a soybean base.

You should not offer plain cow's milk before six months of age, since babies fed on whole milk in the early months of life sometimes suffer from severe gastrointestinal problems. And you should not offer skim milk until your child is over two years. It may not provide the necessary fatty acids that babies need for brain growth and for the development of hormones and enzyme systems. Furthermore, since it is too high in protein concentration for the baby's digestive system to handle easily, it can cause dehydration.

A baby who's several months old before being offered a bottle will probably be mystified by the strange contraption the first time around, and may absolutely refuse to try sucking the rubber nipple. If you plan to wean your baby before six to eight months of age, you should begin offering an occasional bottle at about six to eight weeks of age, to let him get used to this way of getting food. If your baby absolutely refuses a bottle, you may have to feed him by using a teaspoon or cup.

When your baby is about five months of age, you can begin offering a few sips of milk from a cup. By the time she's really ready for it, she'll be quite proficient at draining it to the last drop.

If you have a family history of allergy, avoid cow's milk as long as possible. The later a baby is given a potentially allergenic food, the less likely he is to react against it. Don't try formula until about six months, and then watch your baby closely. If he vomits, gets diarrhea, or shows other unusual reactions, don't give any milk other than breast milk and be careful about any other additions to the diet.

Water and Juice

While breastfed babies don't *need* water, even in hot and dry climates, some enjoy it. If you want to give your baby an occasional bottle of water *after* breastfeeding is well established, there's no harm in it.

Some babies like fruit juice, which can be offered in a bottle if you want to anytime after three months of age. It isn't necessary, though, and if you have a family history of allergy, you may want to wait until after six, or even eight months of age, to lower the chances of your baby's developing an allergy to fruit.

Solid Foods

Breast milk is an ideal total food for the young infant but older babies need additional foods to meet their growing nutritional requirements. Sometime between four and eight months of age, you'll want to start giving your baby solid foods. Advantages to starting on the early side—between four and six months—include the ability to provide iron fortification in cereal, the openness to new experiences that are more characteristic of younger rather than older babies, and the extra time your baby will have to learn how to handle these new foods before she needs them for nourishment.

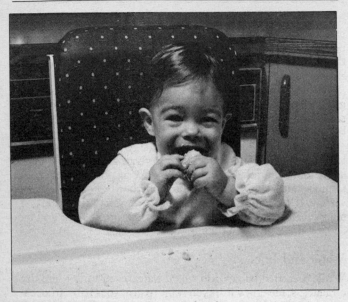

*A chewy unseeded bagel makes a good early
finger food, as this little girl's smile shows.*

Some years ago mothers were advised to begin feeding
their babies solid foods when they were only a couple of weeks
old. We now know that this is not only unnecessary, but un-
wise (as well as a waste of time and money). Such foods may
strain a baby's immature digestive system. Furthermore, they
can fill a baby up so much that she doesn't nurse as vigorously
or becomes too fat, or they may predispose a baby to allergies.

How, then, will you know when to offer your baby solid
foods? Look for signs of readiness in the baby. First, he should
be able to sit up with support, at least in an infant seat, and
should have good control of the head and neck muscles. This
way, he'll be able to show you when he wants food by leaning
forward and opening his mouth, and to show when he doesn't
by leaning back and turning away. If he can't do this, pushing
food into his mouth will constitute a kind of forced feeding.

Nurse your baby first before you offer her food by spoon.
She'll be more open to trying a new experience if she isn't

wildly hungry. Consider these first few feedings of solids "practice feeds," just like those first few nursings so many months ago. After all, your baby now has to learn how to master a completely new set of muscle movements to take the food from a spoon and to swallow it. At first she'll get more food on her face, her bib, and you than she will in her mouth. You'll be surprised, though, at how quickly she'll catch on, and how soon she'll start eating finger foods.

WHEN SHOULD YOU WEAN FROM THE BREAST?

While you'll probably be asked more times than you care to think about how long you plan to breastfeed, there's no reason why you have to set an advance deadline on the duration of breastfeeding, any more than you set a date well ahead of time for the length of time you plan to wheel your baby in a stroller. You'll stop nursing when the time seems right for both you and your baby.

This is a topic on which many people have strong opinions, but few have any evidence to base them on. There's no single optimal time for weaning, as we can see from the great range of weaning ages around the world. In many countries babies are routinely nursed well into the second or third year of life, while in our society women who nurse babies older than a year are often "closet" nursers, who feel they need to hide what they're doing to avoid having to defend the practice.

During the first couple of days, babies get the immunologic benefits of the colostrum; they continue to receive immunologic benefits from breast milk for months. During the first six months, babies can satisfy *all* their nutritional needs from breast milk; after this time they can get what they need from breast milk or cow's milk and from additional simple foods. By nine months they usually have enough teeth and the intestinal maturity to handle a wide variety of foods. They're still, of course, dependent on their parents for many of the essentials of life, but from a nutritional aspect, they need not be dependent on their mother's milk.

The emotional benefit that mother and baby derive from

breastfeeding are just as valid, however, at two months, six months, nine months, a year, or later. You're still maintaining a special intimate relationship with your baby, still able to comfort him at your breast when he's sick, unhappy, or in a strange situation. You're still able to forget the cares of the day for those peaceful minutes while the two of you are a nursing couple.

If you want to continue nursing for emotional reasons rather than for nutritional ones, there's no need to stop at any specified time. On the other hand, if you decide to stop nursing after three months, you need not feel apologetic. Even if you have nursed for only a few weeks and you have to or want to stop breastfeeding, you are still a successful nursing mother. You've given your baby a good start in life and you have known the special joy of the nursing relationship. A little breastfeeding is better than none at all.

How, then, do you decide when to wean? You and your baby together constitute the nursing couple; either one of you may begin the process. Under baby-led weaning, you continue to nurse until your baby loses interest, which may happen sometime between seven and 10 months. Babies of this age sometimes reject the breast completely and refuse to nurse, no matter how you try to hold their interest. Or they may nurse eagerly for a minute or two and then—just as soon as your milk lets down—pull away, and show no further interest. Or you may have a jolly gymnast on your hands (and your lap)—a baby who starts to stand up and flex her muscles while nursing. Babies who act in these ways are often letting their mothers know that they're ready to say good-bye to their nursing days. If a baby hasn't led the way toward weaning by 18 months, he's apt to become so attached to nursing and so identified in his own mind as a nursing child that he's not likely to think about weaning himself for another year or two. If you want to initiate weaning, it's wise to do so before the age of 18 months.

Suppose that your baby or toddler has shown no signs of giving up the breast, but you are restless. The baby eagerly takes an occasional bottle, eats healthy portions of solid food, and drinks from a cup. You have gone back to work or resumed other activities. You look at your nursling and, with some annoyance, wonder, "Is he ever going to stop?"

At this point you have options. You can continue to

nurse, accepting the fact that your baby still benefits from the experience and making efforts to be more patient. But if you find yourself resenting your nursing child you may be doing both of you a favor by taking a gentle initiative toward weaning. Otherwise, your baby will sense your annoyance and impatience. It's better for a baby to drink a bottle happily than to nurse at a grudging breast, just as it's better for a baby to be cared for by a warm, affectionate baby-sitter than by a restless, unhappy mother who would rather be at work.

On the other hand, suppose you would really like to continue breastfeeding past your child's first, second, or even third birthday, but are embarrassed by the idea. (Somehow friends, relatives, and perfect strangers criticize a late nurser more than they do the toddler or preschooler who carries a bottle around.) You may wonder whether late nursing may make a child too dependent. There's no evidence that it does. Children who were nursed as toddlers don't seem to be any different from children who were weaned earlier. Provided the mother-child relationship is warm and loving, the length of

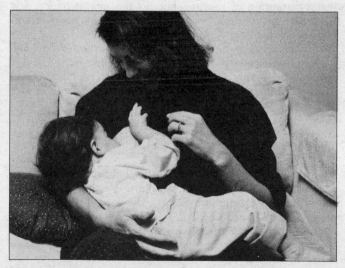

There's no "right age" to wean a baby; nursing is good as long as both mother and child want it to continue.

breastfeeding—or even the fact of breastfeeding itself—does not seem to be an all-important factor in a child's healthy psychological development.

One problem that your child may encounter if he is still nursing at a later age than is typical in our society is teasing or ridicule from relatives, neighbors, or even strangers. If this happens, you can speak to the persons doing the teasing, asking them to talk to you and not your child about any feelings they have about the appropriateness of your child's nursing. You can also speak to your child directly, reassuring him that you feel it is perfectly fine for him to continue nursing, but that some other people don't understand how important this is to children. You can also give him the option of nursing in private, to avoid public comment. If he wants to give up nursing, you can let him know that this is fine with you, that this is a decision he can certainly make.

If possible, try to initiate weaning at a time when your baby does not have to make other adjustments. If she's teething or has a cold, or you've just gone back to work, or there's a new baby-sitter, or you've just moved, or there's some other major disruption of routine, put off the weaning for a few weeks. It's always easier for children (and adults, too) to manage one change at a time.

Whatever your choice, when people ask you, "What? *Still* nursing?" or exclaim, "You gave up *already*?" feel free to answer that you think this a decision every nursing couple needs to make for itself and that you feel that this is the best choice for you.

HOW SHOULD YOU WEAN?

There may not be a right time to wean, but there is definitely a right way—gradually, sympathetically, and with a positive attitude. Weaning is a natural process; the natural way to help it along is to do it little by little, over a period of some weeks. Weaning represents a positive growth experience for the two of you. It's a sign that your baby is able to become independent of you in one important way and, as such, is the first step in a series of independent steps. It's best accomplished slowly and gradually. It's worst done "cold turkey," which results in physi-

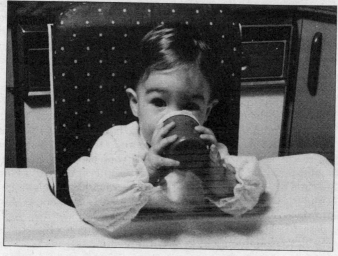

*Holding and drinking from a cup is
one more sign of a developing independence.*

cal pain for you and in emotional pain for both you and your
baby.

Baby-led Weaning

If you're still enjoying the breastfeeding and are in no hurry to
stop, but feel that weaning would be appropriate at this time in
your child's life, you can let your nursing child lead the way.
One phrase that governs the process for many mothers is
"Don't offer; don't refuse." This way, you nurse when your
child asks to, but don't suggest it at other times. While it
sometimes seems hard to believe, even the most eager nurser
will eventually find other activities and foods and comforts
that are more interesting than nursing. With an older child,
the end of nursing sometimes happens so gradually that you
may not even think of it as weaning. One day you may suddenly realize it's been several days since you've nursed. Typi-
cally, your child may ask to nurse a few more times, but by that
time you may have no milk and the charm will be gone. Still a
loving couple, you're no longer a nursing couple.

Some mothers accelerate this process in various ways. One, for example, told her three-year-old that if she was old enough to chew gum, she was too old to nurse. The little girl was not about to give up her sugar-free bubble gum and never asked to nurse again. Another mother told her three-year-old a story about a little rabbit whose mother said, "I love you and love to nurse you, but my milk is going away and it's really special milk for babies." Other mothers vary their children's routines with substitutes like a game, a cuddle, a walk to the park, a reading session with a favorite book, or a piece of fruit or other healthful snack. Most important is your involvement with the activity, so that you show your baby that you can show your love for him in many ways. Others find that asking a child to postpone a nursing will sometimes lead to his forgetting it. A child who asks to nurse in public, for example, can often accept waiting "until we get home." Sometimes he'll dash inside to collect what's been promised; at other times he'll become interested in something else.

Mother-led Weaning

If you're ready to wean, but your baby hasn't shown any sign of losing interest, you may want to start the ball rolling yourself.

First pinpoint the nursing session your baby shows the least interest in. It will probably be the early evening or noon-time feeding. Eliminate this one first. If your baby is under a year old, substitute a bottle. Most babies enjoy sucking on a bottle until they're well past a year, but not all find them appealing. If your baby doesn't seem interested, don't try to force a bottle on him. Instead, substitute something else, like a cup of juice or a few spoonfuls of applesauce.

Wait several days, up to two weeks, and then eliminate the next lightest feeding of the day. Keep doing this until you're down to one nursing a day, probably the first one of the morning or the last one at night. By now, you'll be producing very little milk and your baby may give up this last feeding easily. Or you may decide to continue this one favorite feeding for a while longer. Weaning this way should take from a couple of weeks to a couple of months or longer.

If you wean slowly like this, you should have little or no discomfort from milk pressure. You'll gradually produce less and less milk until there's virtually none at all. If at any point during weaning, your breasts become overfull, you can express just enough milk to ease your discomfort or put your baby to the breast for a minute or two (if she's willing to stop at that). Don't overdo it or you'll just encourage your breasts to continue producing copious amounts of milk. If you're uncomfortably full most of the time, slow down the weaning process.

Make yourself as available to your baby as possible during the weaning. Since she's losing something she has valued greatly—the pleasure of suckling at your breast—she needs the reassurance of your love and comforting. If you can devote extra time to her now, this should be reassuring. While you don't need to feel guilty or apologetic, you do want to recognize the adjustment she's making and help her make it more smoothly through your loving understanding. Weaning seems to be fairly easy for babies under a year; after this time the child develops an attachment that is harder to change, and the mother needs to be more patient. For suggestions on weaning the older nursing child, see the box on the following page (Weaning the Older Child).

Sudden Weaning

Sometimes a situation comes up that requires abrupt weaning—a serious illness of the mother, perhaps, or some other emergency. If you absolutely have to wean suddenly, you'll probably be uncomfortable for several days unless you have been producing very little milk. You can relieve your discomfort by expressing just enough milk to ease the pressure on your breasts. You might also ask your doctor to prescribe medication that is effective in preventing lactation. And you may also get relief from hot compresses.

YOUR FEELINGS ABOUT WEANING

When you stop breastfeeding, your body will undergo a number of physiological changes as your hormonal balance reverts to what it was before you became pregnant. The most obvious change will be in your breasts. It may take three or four

Weaning the Older Child

•Make an agreement with your child about the places that nursing can take place. For example, only at home, in the car, or in a friend's house, but not in a restaurant or other public place.

•Make the nursing sessions shorter.

•Use distraction. Before a child might ordinarily nurse or as you're bringing a short nursing session to an end, involve her in an interesting activity.

•Offer something your child likes to eat just before he would ordinarily nurse.

•Change your usual routine. At a usual nursing time, go out for a walk or a ride, or invite a playmate over, or bring out a new toy.

•Stay away from the places where you ordinarily nurse. If you're used to nursing in a special chair, maybe you can move it out of your home temporarily.

•Do not uncover your breasts in front of your child. This will remind him of nursing.

•Give your child a lot of physical affection in activities not associated with breastfeeding, such as reading a picture book, telling stories, or singing.

months for you to lose all of your milk, even though none may be apparent within days after the last nursing session. It may also take several months for your breasts to return to their former size. They will most likely be less firm than they were before you became pregnant, but this is the result of childbearing, not breastfeeding. They'll probably seem to be the same size they were before your pregnancy, although some women feel that their breasts become larger or smaller after nursing. This may have something to do with the amount of weight

•Enlist the child's favorite people. Ask your husband to put her to bed, to go to her in the middle of the night, to rock and cuddle her.

•Focus on eliminating the nursing sessions that are most inconvenient for you and let the others continue for a while.

•Talk to your child about weaning as a definite occurrence in the future (after the next birthday, perhaps, or after Santa Claus comes). Even if there's some backsliding after these events, your child will think of nursing as ending someday.

•Emphasize what a big boy or girl your child is. Focus on the many things he can do for himself, like dressing himself, going to the potty, and going to nursery school. Talk about nursing as something that's important for little children but not for big ones.

•While you're weaning, continue to be willing to nurse your child at times when she's especially needy. If she hurts herself or is sick or unhappy, depriving her of the comfort she's used to will only create more unhappiness for both of you. Once she's weaned, you'll be able to comfort her in other ways.

•Don't resort to traumatic techniques like painting your breasts with pepper, soot, or evil-tasting substances. Allow your child to keep his happy memories and his trust in you.

gained or lost or with their having become accustomed to having larger breasts.

Your emotional reactions to weaning may be even more apparent than your physical responses. If your baby is setting the pace for weaning earlier than you had expected, you may be feeling rejected. Rejoice, instead, in your child's push for independence and in his demonstration that he can take the initiative toward a new chapter in his life.

While it can be a blow to realize that your child does not

need you in this particular way as much as she did before, you shouldn't lose sight of the fact that she'll need you even more in other ways. Right now, for example, she may have special needs for the comfort of your arms and the reassurance of your love. Parenthood involves learning what our children need at different stages in their lives—and being willing to give it.

Even if you yourself initiate the weaning process, you may be surprised to find that you feel more than a little sad as nursing draws to a close. The end of breastfeeding represents a loss to you both. No longer will you enjoy this close physical bond, this symbiosis between you and your baby in which you needed each other in a very special way. The end of nursing, especially of a long-time nursing relationship, marks the beginning of a new phase in your child's life. And as much as we want our children to grow up and be independent, most of us have ambivalent feelings about the results of our success. You'll probably have the same kind of mixed emotions the first time you leave each of your children playing happily in preschool or kindergarten. A lump in the parental throat often accompanies our feelings of accomplishment for having helped our children to meet life's challenges with confidence and enthusiasm.

STAYING CLOSE WITH YOUR CHILD

When you wean your baby and help her take this first big step toward independence, you will very likely look back over her young life. You think of the months you carried her under your heart, nourishing her through your body. You remember the exertion on both your parts as she burst into the world as an individual human being, breathing through her own lungs, making her own efforts to draw nourishment, learning how to cope with a strange world. You dwell on the time you spent together as a nursing couple, reliving the many happy moments you knew as you held your baby in your arms and gave deeply of yourself.

And then you look forward. You think of the many other ways you will give of yourself to this child: the guidance you will provide to help him find his way in life, the love that will

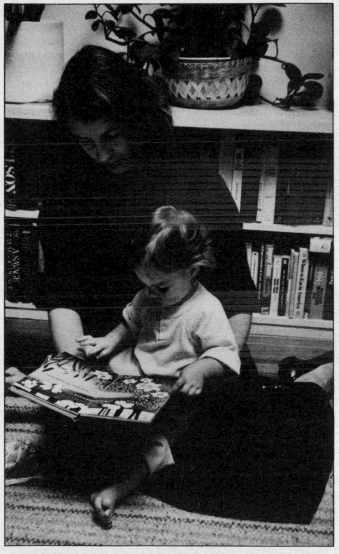

After breastfeeding has stopped, mothers and their children will continue to enjoy doing many other things together.

support him, the courage you will give him to let go of you and be his own person, the happy hours you'll spend enjoying each other's company, playing together, having fun. You accept the fact that as a mother you will know tears and anger, as well as laughter and delight. But just as you now remember, not the minor setbacks or worries about breastfeeding, but its heartfelt joys, so too will you balance out the stresses and demands of motherhood with the love and the warmth and the personal growth that you gain from your relationship with your children.

Appendix

Expressing, Storing, and Offering Breast Milk

Throughout this book we talk about situations in which you might want to express your milk to give to your baby. This Appendix provides practical, "how-to" suggestions that have worked for other nursing mothers, which you can adapt for yourself. For special recommendations for working nursing mothers, see Chapter 9.

EXPRESSING MILK

There are several ways of expressing milk—by hand, by manual pump, and by electric pump. The method you decide on will depend on your own individual needs and preferences, based on your own unique situation, as well as on comfort, convenience, and economy. We'll describe the different methods here—and then go on to discuss storage and ways of offering your milk.

Some of the principles that apply to all methods include the following:

Cleanliness. Before you express by any method, wash your hands with soap and water, bathe or wipe off your breasts with a moistened cloth (no soap, alcohol, or other drying agents), and be sure your equipment is clean. (See the section on "Containers" in this chapter.)

It takes time and practice to master all the methods. If you can plan ahead (as, for example, for going back to work), practice at home for a while before you need to express regularly. If you don't get the amount of milk you'd like at first, keep it up.

Some Ways to Enhance Milk Production When Expressing

You may want to try one or more of the following methods to increase your flow of milk. Different methods are effective for different women.

•Prop a photo of your baby in front of you. Look at it and remember what it feels like (or imagine what it will feel like) to have him at your breast. (Or use a photo of you nursing the baby.)

•Visualize your baby in your mind. Imagine what she looks like, sounds like, feels like, smells like when she nurses.

•For two to five minutes before you begin, do deep breathing or some other relaxation exercise.

•Make yourself as comfortable as possible.

•If your surroundings permit, sit with your feet up.

•Just before you begin, lay a warm towel on your breast for a minute or two. Then massage the breast gently, starting from the top and moving around the sides and the bottom, moving your fingers in a circular motion. Stroke yourself lightly from the armpit, from above and below the breast, and from the middle of the chest toward the nipple. You don't need to massage or stroke the nipples themselves. (You can massage your breasts even while you're dressed.)

The more you do it, the more efficient you'll become, and the more milk you'll yield.

The first time you express, try to choose a quiet time when you're not likely to be distracted or interrupted. Also, give yourself as much help as you can. Ask someone to be with you, if possible someone who's done it herself. It's wonderful to have someone to answer the telephone or doorbell, take care of an older child, provide another pair of hands in any way you need them. Then get yourself comfortable—in a chair or couch, with pillows for support. And do whatever you can to

---

•Lean over and shake your breasts gently.

•Drink a cup of hot tea. If your baby is not sensitive to cow's milk products that you eat or drink, you might try warm milk or cocoa.

•Switch breasts at least once during each session and preferably twice, to insure maximum emptying. Usually the second expression of each breast is briefer than the first.

•Make the time go faster by talking with a friend, listening to the radio, reading, or watching television while you're expressing or pumping.

•If your baby is present but cannot suck and if you don't need two hands to express, hold him while you're pumping.

•Wear comfortable clothes that open up or pull up but still cover your shoulders, so you don't get chilled.

•Listen to music that you associate with nursing. This works best if you play the record initially during actual breastfeeding sessions; then when you're expressing, hearing the same music may help evoke the memory and the sensations you felt then. (Handel's "Water Music" gets high marks from some women who enjoy classical music.)

•If you're having a lot of trouble getting started, you may want to ask your doctor to prescribe an oxytocin nasal spray that you can use on a temporary basis. Note, though, that if used for longer than a week or more often than twice a day it loses its effectiveness.

relax. The suggestions above may help you enhance your milk production.

Effect of time of day. Since most women's milk supply tends to drop at about 6 P.M., you'll probably have greater success if you express earlier in the day. (Between 7 A.M. and 1 P.M. is the best time for the first sessions; late afternoon and early evening are the worst.) Working women often find that their milk supply diminishes during the week, so that by Friday they're giving less than they did on Monday, when they had the weekend to take things a little easier. Knowing this may help you plan your schedule and accept your body's ability to yield milk.

Expressing while nursing. Several of the methods allow you to take advantage of the ejecting of milk that often flows from one breast while the other is being stimulated. Instead of wasting this milk, or looking on it as a nuisance, you can build your expressing program around it. Another advantage to this method is that it tends to increase your milk supply. This double-duty nursing can fool your body into thinking that you're nursing twins, and operating by the law of supply and demand, it will produce more milk. Specific ways to do this are described under the different methods.

Hand Expression

Manual expression is a valuable skill to have, since you can do it at any time, without any equipment other than your own body and something to catch the milk. Many mothers prefer it above other methods because it's more natural, it allows for skin-to-skin contact and, of course, it doesn't cost anything. It requires practice to become proficient, and some women never get milk from this method. Others get so good at it that they wouldn't express any other way. Here's how to do it:

•Wash your hands.

•Position a clean cup, wide-mouthed jar, or thermos under your breast.

•Hold your breast with your thumb above and your first two fingers below, about an inch or an inch and a half behind the nipple. For most women this is the edge of the areola, but if your areola is narrower or wider, it's the distance that counts.

•Push your thumb and fingers together, back toward the chest wall.

•Gently roll the thumb and fingers forward to empty the milk pools.

•Repeat the push-roll sequence a few times until no more drops come out.

•Do this at several different spots around the breast. Some positions may be better for you than others.

•Do not squeeze or cup the breast, slide your fingers, or pull out the skin on the breast.

•Be sure the milk does not run over your index finger as it flows.

•If you don't get any milk the first few times, keep trying.

Milk Cups

By using milk cups[1] (also called breast shields or shells) that don't have holes in the outer shell, you can collect milk from one breast as you're nursing or pumping on the other, thus taking advantage of normal leakage and not wasting a drop of milk.

•This method is helpful for working mothers or others who'll be giving their milk within a short time to healthy, full-term babies. It is not advisable when expressing milk for a premature or sick baby or for donation to a milk bank.

•As you're nursing or expressing on one breast, wear a *sterilized*

---

[1]These can be purchased from maternity shops, drugstores, or childbirth education organizations, including La Leche League.

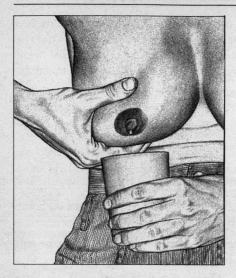

Women who become skillful at expressing milk by hand usually prefer it to any other method.

milk cup in your bra on the other. When the cup fills, empty it into a clean bottle. You may have to empty it more than once during a feeding if you have a strong let-down.

•When you finish nursing or expressing on the first breast, refrigerate the milk in the bottle.

•Do not wear the milk-filled cup longer than 15 minutes, since the warmth from your body may encourage the growth of bacteria. Do not use milk that collects between feedings.

•At the next feeding, start with the other breast and wear a clean, newly sterilized milk cup on the first side. Repeat this procedure.

Hand-held Pump

There are several different kinds of pumps available, and more are being developed constantly. To find the one you like the best, ask other women what kinds they've tried and which ones they're happy with. See whether you can borrow different models, either from a friend who isn't using theirs at the moment, or from a local hospital, lactation consultant, childbirth education group, or La Leche League chapter. Decide which features are important for you and evaluate the pumps you see based on your own needs. Take the time to read the instructions that come with the pump.

Some of the most important features to look for are:

•*Gentleness:* It should not hurt.

•*Effectiveness:* It should empty the breast almost as well as the baby does and stimulate further production of milk, and it should do this fairly quickly.

•*Safety:* It should be easy to clean so that bacteria do not accumulate to spoil the milk.

•*Portability:* If you plan to carry the pump to and from work, it should be easy to carry.

•*Convenience:* It's better if it doesn't have too many separate parts.

Kinds of Pumps Available

As of this writing, the following pumps are available and the following evaluations are based on research, professional opinion, and the comments of women who have used them. Prices are likely to change.

•**Bulb-type.** These small "bicycle horn" pumps consisting of a glass cup attached to a rubber bulb are *not* recommended. They're sold in many drugstores and are the least expensive kind (about $6), but are generally unsatisfactory for several reasons. They're potentially dangerous, because they're so hard to clean that drops of milk cling to them, and mold and bacteria grow. Furthermore, they're hard to use and often uncomfortable since the cup that's supposed to fit over the nipple doesn't press down on the areola. While a few women like this kind, all in all, they're best avoided.

•**Trigger-type.** The Loyd-B is a simple pump shaped like a gun. You put it to the breast and pull a trigger which creates suction on the breast, making the milk flow into a small baby-food jar. You can control the amount of suction by the force you use to squeeze the trigger. While many women like this one, it has drawbacks. Because it requires a fair amount of dexterity, the breast opposite the dominant hand (the left breast for right-handed women) gets emptied more efficiently; thus plugged ducts may develop on the other breast. Also, it's hard to use while you're nursing and women with small hands have difficulty working it. Finally, its glass parts sometimes break and may be hard to replace. It runs about $25.

•**Syringe-type.** This kind of pump is the most popular. It's easy to operate, easy to clean, and easy to carry around. It consists of two cylinders, one of which fits inside the other; the pumping is accomplished by moving the outer cylinder up and down; the piston action creates suction. The end of the smaller cylinder fits over the breast, and milk is collected in the larger cylinder, which can then be fitted with a nipple and used as a feeding bottle.

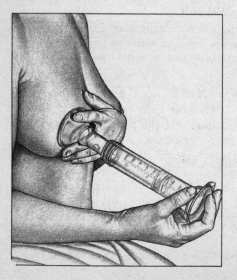

The most popular hand-held pump is the syringe-type, which is available from several different manufacturers.

The most popular pumps of this kind are the Marshall/ Kaneson Breast Pump/Infant Nurser and the Happy Family. Some of the others that have recently come on the market are the Infa, the AXipump, the Breast Pump Kit by Mary Jane, the Nursing Mother Breast Pump by Motherhood Maternity Boutique, the Faultless Deluxe, and the Medela Manual Breastpump/Feeding System. (One advantage of the Medela is that it can also be used in conjunction with an electric pump, so that a woman can switch back and forth between the manual and the electric pump.) These pumps, which are fairly similar, cost from $12 to $30; shopping around (by phone or in person) often pays off.

To pump while nursing, get the baby started first. Prop her on a pillow under the nursing breast. For the first few times, when you're ready to pump ask a helper to hold the baby in position. Then you can use both your hands to work the pump. After you do this several times, you'll get the hang of it and will be able to do it by yourself.

•**Battery-operated.** A couple of manufacturers (Egnell and Healthteam in South Plainfield, New Jersey) have recently introduced battery-operated hand-held pumps. By pressing on a bar, you activate an alternating suction action designed to imitate a baby's sucking. The milk goes into a small nursing bottle that can be refrigerated or frozen. Since these pumps can be operated with one hand, they can be used while nursing. They sell for about $35. They sound like a good idea, but so far these pumps don't fulfill their promise. They provide neither the power of an electric nor the control of the hand-operated pumps, and the alarming rate at which they use up batteries drives up the cost considerably.

•**Electric pump.** Electric pumps are the easiest to use. They're comfortable, efficient, and fast; they automatically control suction to simulate a baby's sucking action; and while they're doing the work you can read, watch television, or do paperwork. Their biggest drawback is expense. Both the Egnell and the Medela, the most popular electric pumps, cost about $1,000, although they can be rented from pharmacies, medical supply houses, hospitals, childbirth education and La

Leche League groups for about $20 a week.[2] The White River and Schuco are less expensive (about $400 and $250) and can also be rented. If you can afford it, it may be worth the expense to rent an electric pump for a while; it's sometimes possible to get a lower price if you contract to rent over a period of several months.

If your doctor prescribes breastfeeding for some medical reason (such as your baby's prematurity or allergy to cow's milk) and if pumping is necessary, your medical insurance may cover the cost. You may be able to join with other nursing mothers to rent one jointly, to keep at your place of work or another central location.

STORING MILK

Containers

The best containers for keeping your breast milk are four-ounce plastic nursing bottles or disposable plastic nurser bags, depending on your preference.

• You want plastic rather than glass for two reasons: First, some research suggests that some of the *leukocytes* (white blood cells) in breast milk cling to glass, making them unavailable to your baby. They cling less to plastic. Second, plastic doesn't break when dropped, and as one nursing mother said, "My milk is liquid gold!"

• You want the small bottles rather than the eight-ounce ones, so that you can defrost small amounts: Babies drink smaller amounts of breast milk than of formula since they digest it more easily, and once thawed, milk should not be refrozen.

• There is some controversy over the use of the disposable plastic bags that fit into nursing bottles. Some research suggests

---

[2]For more information, contact Egnell, Inc., 765 Industrial Drive, Cary, IL 60013 (800) 323-8750; Medela, P.O. Box 386, Crystal Lake, IL 60014 (800) 435-8316; White River, c/o Elena Grant, 10250 Southwest 130 Ave., Beaverton, OR 97005; Schuco, Division of ACI, P.O. Box 246, 201 Hillside Ave., Williston Park, NY 11596 (516) 741-7110.

that secretory IgA (an important immunity-conferring component of human milk) becomes unavailable to the baby by being stored in such bags, but there is a difference of opinion in
the medical community about the validity of such findings.
The bags need careful handling to avoid spillage and puncture, they sometimes split when frozen, and they absorb odors
from nearby foods; on the other hand they thaw faster and are
easier to store than the bottles.

Cleaning and Sterilizing

If you're collecting milk to be given to your own baby within
48 hours, you don't need to sterilize your bottles, nipples, and
pumping equipment. Wash everything thoroughly with a bottle brush and nipple brush to remove any milk scum, and then
wash in a dishwasher or a basin of hot soapy water. Be sure to
rinse all the soap out.

If you are going to take milk to the hospital for a sick or
premature baby or for donation to a milk bank, or if you want
to freeze it for your own future use, you should sterilize your
containers and equipment. If you have a dishwasher that uses
water at 180° F, this will sterilize everything well enough.
Otherwise, do the following: To sterilize just a few things, pad
the inside of a large pot and fill it with enough water to completely cover the items you're sterilizing (such as bottles, cup,
bottle caps, nipples, and funnel). Bring the water to a boil over
high heat; then turn down the heat just enough so that water
continues to boil gently. After five minutes of boiling, remove
the nipples with sterile tongs. Place them on a clean towel.
Allow the other items to boil for 15 minutes longer. Do not
touch the rims of the bottles or the insides of the caps.

Storage

For use within 30 minutes: Give to your baby; no special storage is needed.

For use within six hours: Pour into a clean container; cap
tightly; refrigerate. If refrigeration is impossible, sterilize the
container.

For use within 48 hours: Refrigerate at 40° F (4° C).

For use within one to two weeks: Pour into a sterile container; quick-cool in the refrigerator for 30 minutes; then freeze in refrigerator-freezer unit.

For use within six months: Quick-cool in the refrigerator for 30 minutes. Then freeze at 0° F (−18° C) or below in the freezer of a two-door refrigerator or a deep freeze. (Check temperature with a freezer thermometer at different places in the unit. If your freezer does not get this cold but does keep frozen foods hard, keep the milk in the center of the freezer and use within three months. Frost-free refrigerators, which have a warming element, generally don't maintain 0°.)

It's probably not a good idea to plan on keeping frozen breast milk for longer than this. While instructions are sometimes given for keeping frozen milk up to two years, long-term freezing alters the chemical composition of the milk. (Some of the fats break down, and the milk loses some of its ability to fight harmful organisms.) Furthermore, you run the risk of contamination if you lose electrical power and the milk thaws and refreezes.

Guidelines

•Label each container of frozen milk with the date.

•Don't fill bottles or bags to the top. Milk expands as it freezes, so no more than three and a half ounces should go into a four-ounce bottle.

•You can collect milk a little at a time, chill it in the refrigerator, and add the cold milk to milk that's already frozen. It will have an interesting layered look that will not affect its quality. Be sure to chill the milk first; adding warm milk can defrost the top layer of the frozen milk.

•You can also freeze milk in a plastic ice-cube tray covered by plastic wrap. The frozen cubes (about half an ounce to an ounce each, depending on the size of the compartments) can then be transferred to an airtight plastic or glass container.

When you or your sitter is ready to feed your baby, put the number of cubes you need in a feeding bottle and defrost. This way you have more flexibility, since you can defrost only what your baby needs.

TRANSPORTING EXPRESSED MILK

Keep the milk cold, whether it's refrigerated or frozen. You can do this whatever way is most convenient for you—in a thermos, in an insulated bottle bag, in an ice chest, in an insulated bag filled with cubes, or in ice-packs. Check the method you're using to be sure that refrigerated milk is still cold when it arrives at its destination and that frozen milk is still frozen. If frozen milk has started to thaw, refrigerate it immediately and use within 12 hours.

OFFERING EXPRESSED MILK

Defrosting and Feeding

•Avoid overnight thawing of milk.

•Do not leave out at room temperature.

•Do not try to thaw frozen milk on top of the stove—it will curdle.

•Do not heat either breast milk or formula in a microwave oven. Vitamins are destroyed, and hot spots may occur, which could burn the baby's mouth.

•About half an hour before feeding time take the container from the freezer and hold it under tepid running water. Gradually increase the temperature of the water to hot. Shake the bag or bottle gently, as you warm it; this remixes the cream that has separated. (Since your milk is not homogenized, the fat rises to the top on standing.) This should take only a few minutes. This method can also be used to heat refrigerated milk.

•Do not heat milk on the stove. First, there's a danger of overheating and destroying antibodies and nutrients. Then there's the all-too-common scenario of the mother or baby-sitter warming milk in a pan of water on the stove who runs to answer the phone or the door—and comes back to find the bottle or bag melted and the milk sticking to the bottom of the pan. No way to treat that liquid gold—or the baby waiting for the milk.

•Shake the bottle again before feeding.

•Use milk that has been defrosted but not heated within 12 hours. If the milk has been heated, use within 30 minutes.

•Discard any milk in the bottle that the baby does not finish at one feeding. Trying to give it to your baby later could cause diarrhea.

•Do not refreeze defrosted milk. If you can't use it within the suggested time limit, throw it away.

•If you have both fresh and frozen milk, give your baby the fresh milk and save the frozen for supplements and emergencies.

These measures sound terribly complicated, but most women who express milk for their babies find that once they establish a routine, they are able to carry it off. If it does become too burdensome, it's always possible, of course, to switch to formula. If you do make this switch, don't berate yourself for the change. Instead, congratulate yourself for the efforts you have made and for your contributions to your baby's health and well-being.

Bibliography

Aggett, P. J. (1980, April). Trace elements in human nutrition. *Journal of Tropical Pediatrics*, 43–45.

Ainsworth, M. D. S. and Bell, S. (1977). Infant crying and maternal responsiveness: A rejoinder to Gewirtz & Boyd. *Child Development*, 48, 1208–16.

Alemi, B., Hamosh, M., Scanlon, J. W., Slazman-Mann, C., and Hamosh, P. (1981). Fat digestion in very low-birth-weight infants: Effect of addition of human milk to low-birth-weight formula. *Pediatrics*, 68(4): 484–488.

American Academy of Pediatrics, Committee on Drugs. (1982). Psychotropic drugs in pregnancy and lactation. *Pediatrics*, 69(2): 241–244.

American Academy of Pediatrics, Committee on Drugs. (1983). The transfer of drugs and other chemicals into human breast milk. *Pediatrics*, 72(3): 375–383.

American Academy of Pediatrics, Committee on Nutrition. (1980). On the feeding of supplemental foods to infants. *Pediatrics*, 65(6): 1178–81.

American Academy of Pediatrics, Committee on Nutrition. (1980). Vitamin and mineral supplement needs in normal children in the United States. *Pediatrics*, 66(6): 1015–21.

American Academy of Pediatrics, Committee on Nutrition. (1981). Nutrition and lactation. *Pediatrics*, 68(3): 435–43.

Applebaum, R. M. (1969). *Abreast of the Times*.

Applebaum, R. M. (1970). The modern management of successful breast feeding. *Pediatric Clinics of North America*, 17(1): 203–225.

Arnon, S. S., Damus, K., Thompson, B., Midura, T. F., and Chin, J. (1982). Protective role of human milk against sudden death from infant botulism. *Journal of Pediatrics*, 100, 568–73.

Ashkenazi, A., Levin, S., Idar, D., Ayala, O., Rosenberg, I., and Handzel, Z. (1980). In vitro cell-mediated immunologic assay for cow's milk allergy. *Pediatrics*, 66(3): 399–402.

Auerbach, K. G. (1984). Babies, breasts, and bosses. Providing practical help for the employed breastfeeding mother. In *Breastfeeding and Women Today: Conference Proceedings*. Washington, DC: National Center for Education in Maternal and Child Health, pp. 37–55.

Auerbach, K. G. and Avery, J. L. (1980). Relactation: A study of 366 cases. *Pediatrics*, 65(2): 236–42.

Auerbach, K. G. and Avery, J. L. (1981). Induced lactation: A study of adoptive nursing by 240 women. *American Journal of Diseases of Children*, 135, 340–43.

Auerbach, K. G. and Guss, E. (1984). Maternal employment and breastfeeding: A study of 567 women's experiences. *American Journal of Diseases of Children*, 138, 958–60.

Avery, J. L. (1973). *Induced Lactation*. Athens, TN: Lact-Aid International.

Avery, J. L. (1977). Closet nursing: Symptom of intolerance and forerunner of social change? *Keeping Abreast Journal*, 2, 212. Reprinted as 18-page monograph. Athens, TN: Lact-Aid International.

Avery, J. L. (1983). Relactation and induced lactation. In Riordan, J. *A Practical Guide to Breastfeeding*. St. Louis: C. V. Mosby, pp. 275–93.

Baltimore, R. S., Vecchitto, J. S., and Pearson, H. A. (1978). Growth of escherichia coli and concentration of iron in an infant feeding formula. *Pediatrics*, 62(6): 1072–73.

Barber-Madden, R. and Petschek, M. A. (1984). Breastfeeding and the working mother: Barriers and solutions. Paper presented at the American Public Health Assn. Annual Meetings, Anaheim, CA, Nov. 13.

Bell, S. and Ainsworth, M. D. S. (1972). Infant crying and maternal responsiveness. *Child Development*, 43, 1171–90.

Berger, L. (1981). When should one discourage breast-feeding. *Pediatrics*, 67(2): 300–302.

Berlin, C. M., Jr. (1981). Pharmacologic considerations of drug use in the lactating mother. *Obstetrics and Gynecology*, 58(5): (supplement), 17S–23S.

Bitman, J., Wood, D. L., Mehta, N. R., Hamosh, P., and Hamosh, M. (1984, August 27). Lipid composition of breast milk from mothers of term and preterm infants. Paper presented to American Chemical Society, Beltsville, MD.

Blumstein, P., Ph.D., and Schwartz, P., Ph.D. (1983). *American Couples: Money, Work, Sex*. New York: Wm. Morrow.

Boggs, K. R. and Rau, P. K. (1983, October). Breastfeeding the premature infant. *American Journal of Nursing*, 1437–39.

Borglin, N. and Sandholm, L. (1971) Effect of oral contraceptives on lactation. *Fertility-Sterility*, 22, 39–41.

Bose, C. L., D'Ercole, J., Lester, A. G., Hunter, R. S. and Barrett, J. R. (1981). Relactation by mothers of sick and premature infants. *Pediatrics*, 67(4): 565–69.

Bradley, R. A. (1965). *Husband-coached Childbirth*. New York: Harper & Row.

Brazelton, T. B. (1961). Effect of maternal medication on the neonate and his behavior. *Journal of Pediatrics*, 58, 513–18.

Brazelton, T. B. (1983). *Infants and Mothers: Differences in Development*. New York: Delacorte Press.

Brazelton, T. B., M.D. (1985). *Working and Caring*. Reading, MA: Merloyd Lawrence Books (Addison-Wesley).

Brazerol, W., McPhee, A., Lyon, S., Wu, R., and Tsang, R. C. (1984). Serial UV radiation effects on vitamin D metabolites in blacks and whites. Presented to American Pediatric Society. *Pediatric Research*, 18(4): 191A.

Brody, J. (1979, December 4). New studies explain protective benefits of mother's milk. *New York Times*, C1–C2.

Brusky, D. (1984, February 7). U.S. Dept. of Labor. Cited in Petschek and Barber-Madden.

Butte, N. F., Garza, C., Smith, E. O'B., and Nichols, B. F. (1984). Human milk intake and growth in exclusively breastfed infants. *Journal of Pediatrics*, 104, 187–95.

Byers, T., Graham, S., Rzepka, T., and Marshall, J. (1985). Lactation and breast cancer. Evidence for a negative association in premenopausal women. *American Journal of Epidemiology*, 121(5): 664–74.

Cahill, M. A. (1982). Environmental contaminants in breast milk. Information sheet no. 30. Franklin Park, IL: La Leche League International, Inc.

Cant, A., Marsden, R. A., and Kilshaw, P. J. (1986). Egg and cows' milk hypersensitivity in exclusively breast fed infants with eczema, and detection of egg protein in breast milk. *British Medical Journal*, 291: 932–35.

Carpenter, G. (1981, August). The importance of mother's milk. *Natural History*, 90(8): 6, 12, 14.

Casey, C. E., Walravens, P. A., and Hambidge, K. M. (1981). Availability of zinc: Loading tests with human milk, cow's milk, and infant formulas. *Pediatrics*, 68(3): 394–396.

Chess, S., Thomas, A., and Birch, H. G. (1965) *Your Child Is a Person*. New York: Parallax Publishing.

Clarkson, J. E., Cowan, J. O., and Herbison, G. P. (1984). Jaundice in full term healthy neonates—a population study. *Australian Paediatric Journal*, 20(4): 303–8.

Conner, A. E. (1979). Elevated levels of sodium and chloride in milk from mastitic breast. *Pediatrics*, 63(6): 910–11.

Cooperstock, M., Steffen, E., Yolken, R., and Onderdonk, A. (1982). Clostridium difficile in normal infants and sudden infant death syndrome: An association with infant formula feedings. *Pediatrics*, 70(1): 91–95.

Corcoran, A. and Christensen, S. (1985, July 27). Breastfeeding during pregnancy and breastfeeding siblings who aren't twins. Workshop given at La Leche League International Conference, Washington, DC.

Cunningham, A. S. (1979). Morbidity in breast-fed and artificially fed infants. II. *The Journal of Pediatrics*, 95(5): 685–89.

Cushing, A. H. and Anderson, L. (1982). Diarrhea in breast-fed and non-breast-fed infants. *Pediatrics*, 70(6): 921–925.

DeCarvalho, M., et al. (1984, summer). Does the duration and frequency of early breastfeeding affect nipple pain? *Birth*, 11:2.

DeCarvalho, M., Klaus, M., and Merkatz, M. (1982). Frequency of breastfeeding and serum bilirubin concentration. *American Journal of Diseases of Children*, 136: 737–38.

DeCarvalho, M., Robertson, S., Friedman, A., and Klaus, M. (1983). Effect of frequent breastfeeding on early milk production and infant weight gain. *Pediatrics*, 72(3): 307–311.

Devereux, W. P. (1970). Management of mastitis. *American Journal of Obstetrics and Gynecology*, 108, 78–81.

Duncan, B., Schaefer, C., Sibley, B., and Fonseca, N. M. (1984). Reduced growth velocity in exclusively breast-fed infants. *American Journal of Diseases of Children*, 138(3): 309–13.

Dunkle, L. M., Schmidt, R. R. and O'Connor, D. M. (1979). Neonatal herpes simplex infection possibly acquired via maternal breast milk. *Pediatrics*, 63: 250–51.

Dunn, J. and Kendrick, C. (1982). *Siblings: Love, Envy and Understanding*. Cambridge, MA: Harvard University Press.

Dusdieker, L. B., Booth, B. M., Stumbo, P. J., and Eichenberger, J. M. (1985, February). Effect of supplemental fluids on human milk production. *Journal of Pediatrics*, 207–11.

Eastman, P. (1984, May). Your body's biochemical balance. *Self*, 130–32.

Edidin, D. V., Levitsky, L. L., Schey, W., Dumbovic, N., and Campos, A. (1980). Resurgence of nutritional rickets associated with breast-feeding and special dietary practices. *Pediatrics*, 65(2): 232–35.

Eiger, M. S., Rausen, A. R., and Silverio, J. (1984). Breast- vs. bottle-feeding. *Clinical Pediatrics*, 23(9): 492–95.

Errors in babies' food. (1969, November 29). *British Medical Journal*, 515–16.

Fallot, M. E., Boyd, J. L. III, and Oski, F. A. (1980). Breast-feeding reduces incidence of hospital admissions for infection in infants. *Pediatrics*, 65(6): 1121–24.

FAS Reports. (1982, November). The secret of mother's milk. p. 2.

Ferris, A. G., Beal, V. A., Laus, M. J., and Hosmer, D. W. (1979). The effect of feeding on fat deposition in early infancy. *Pediatrics*, 64(4): 397–401.

Filer, L. J., Jr. (1971). Infant feeding in the nineteen seventies. *Pediatrics*, 47, 489–90.

Filsinger, E. E., Fabes, R. A. (1985). Odor communication, pheromones, and human families. *Journal of Marriage and the Family*, 47(2): 349–56.

Finberg, L. (1981). Human milk, feeding and vitamin D supplementation—1981. *Journal of Pediatrics*, 99(2): 228–29.

Fischman, S. H., Raskin, P. H., and Raskin, E. A. (1983). Changes in intimate and sexual relationships in postpartum couples. Presentation given at conference of The Society for the Scientific Study of Sex, Eastern Region, Philadelphia, April 15.

Fisher, W. and Gray, J. (1983, November 18). "Erotophobia-Erotophilia and Couples' Sexual Behavior during Pregnancy and after Childbirth," paper presented at annual meeting of The Society for the Scientific Study of Sex, Chicago.

Folley, S. J. (1956). *The Physiology and Biochemistry of Lactation* London: Oliver and Boyd.

Folley, S. J. (1969). The milk-ejection reflex: a neuroendocrine theme in biology, myth and art. *Journal of Endocrinology*, 44.

Fomon, S. J., Filer, L. J., Jr., Anderson, T. A., and Ziegler, E. E. (1979). Recommendations for feeding normal infants. *Pediatrics*, 63(1): 52–63.

Forman, M. R., Graubard, B. I., Hoffman, H. J., Beren, R., Harley, E. E., and Bennett, P. (1984, December). The Pima infant feeding study: Breast feeding and respiratory infections during the first year of life. Paper accepted by *International Journal of Epidemiology*.

Forman, M. R., Graubard, B. I., Hoffman, H. J., Beren, R., Harley, E. E., and Bennett, P. (1984). The Pima infant feeding study: Breast feeding and gastroenteritis in the first year of life. *American Journal of Epidemiology*, 119(3): 335–49.

Frank, A., Taber, L. H., Glezen, W. P., Kasel, G. L., Wells, C. R., and Paredes, A. (1982). Breast-feeding and respiratory virus infection. *Pediatrics*, 70(2): 239–45.

Frantz, K. B. (1980). Techniques for successfully managing nipple problems and the reluctant nurser in the early postpartum period. In *Human Milk: Its Biological and Social Value*, ed. S. Frier and A. Eidelman, pp. 314–17. *Excerpta Medica*.

Frantz, K. B., Fleiss, P. M., and Lawrence, R. A. (1978). Management of the slow-gaining breastfed baby. *Keeping Abreast Journal*, 3: 287.

Gansberg, J. M. and Mostel, A. P., M. D. (1984). *The Second Nine Months*. New York: Pocket Books.

Gartner, L. M. and Arias, I. M. (1966). Studies of prolonged neonatal jaundice in the breast-fed infant. *Journal of Pediatrics*, 68, 54–66.

Gartner, L. M., Lee, K. S., and Moscioni, A. D. (1983). Effect of milk feeding on intestinal bilirubin absorption in the rat. *Journal of Pediatrics*, 103(3): 464–71.

Gaull, G. E., Wright, C. E., and Isaacs, C. E. (1985). Significance of growth modulators in human milk. *Supplement: Current Issues in Feeding the Normal Infant, Pediatrics*, 75(1, part 2): 142–45.

Gerrard, J. W. and Shenassa, M. (1983). Food allergy: Two common types as seen in breast and formula fed babies. *Annals of Allergy*, 50: 375–79.

Gerrard, J. W. and Shenassa, M. (1983). Sensitization to substances in breast milk: Recognition, management and significance. *Annals of Allergy*, 51: 300–2.

Gillin, F. D., Reiner, D. S., and Gault, M. J. (1985). Cholate-dependent killing of giardia lamblia by human milk. *Infection and Immunity*, 47(3): 619–22.

Gillin, F. D., Reiner, D. S., and Wang, C. S. (1983). Human milk kills parasitic intestinal protozoa. *Science*, 221(4167): 1290–92.

Gioiosa, R. (1955). Incidence of pregnancy during lactation in 500 cases. *American Journal of Obstetrics and Gynecology*, 70, 162.

Goldberg, N. M. and Adams, E. (1983). Supplementary water for breast-fed babies in a hot and dry climate—not really a necessity. *Archives of Diseases of Children*, 58(1): 73–74.

Grams, M. (1985). *Breastfeeding Success for Working Mothers*. Sheridan, WY: Achievement Press.

Grantham-McGregor, S. M. and Back, E. H. (1970). Breast feeding in Kingston, Jamaica. *Archives of Diseases of Children*, 45: 404–9.

Gray, H. F. R. S. (1966). *Anatomy of the Human Body*. 28th Edition. Philadelphia: Lea and Febiger.

Greer, F. R., Hollis, B. W., Cripps, D. J., and Tsang, R. C. (1984). Effects of maternal ultraviolet-B irradiation on the vitamin D content of human milk. *Journal of Pediatrics*, 105(3): 431–33.

Gross, S. J., Geller, J., and Tomarelli, R. M. (1981). Composition of breast milk from mothers of preterm infants. *Pediatrics*, 68(4): 490–93.

Grulee, C. G. and Sanford, H. N. (1936). The influence of breast and artificial feeding on infantile eczema. *Journal of Pediatrics*, 9: 223.

Gruskay, F. L. (1982, August). Comparison of breast, cow, and soy feedings in the prevention of onset of allergic disease: A 15-year prospective study. *Clinical Pediatrics*, 486–491.

György, P. (1971, August). Biochemical aspects, in symposium. The uniqueness of human milk. *American Journal of Clinical Nutrition*, pp. 970–975.

Haagensen, C. D. (1965). Breast feeding and breast disease. *Journal of the American Medical Women's Association*, 20: 956.

Haessler, H. and Harris, R. (1980). *The bodyworkbook*. New York: Avon.

Haire, D. and Haire, J. I. (1971). *The Nurse's Contribution to Successful Breast-Feeding, II. The Medical Value of Breast-Feeding*. Bellevue, WA: International Childbirth Education Association.

Hamberg, L. (1971). Controlled trial of fluoride in vitamin drops for the prevention of caries in children, *Lancet*, 1: 441–42.

Hamosh, M., Bitman, J., Wood, D. L., Hamosh, P. and Mehta, N. R. (1985). Lipids in milk and the first steps in their digestion. *Supplement: Current Issues in Feeding the Normal Infant, Pediatrics*, 75(1, part 2): 146–50.

Hanson, L. A., Ahlstedt, S., Andersson, B., Cruz, J. R., et al. (1984). The immune response of the mammary gland and its significance for the neonate. *Annals of Allergy*, 53(6, Part 2): 576–82.

Hanson, L. A., Ahlstedt, S., Andersson, B., Carlsson, B., Fallstrom, S. P., Porras, L. M. O., Soderstrom, T., and Eden, C. S. (1985). Protective factors in milk and the development of the immune system. *Supplement: Current Issues in Feeding the Normal Infant, Pediatrics*, 75(1, part 2): 172–76.

Harris, B. P. (1969, May 17). Cancer of the breast and lactation. *Canadian Medical Association Journal*, 100: 917.

Hatcher, R. A., Guest, F., Stewart, F., Stewart, G., Trussell, J., Cerel, S., and Cates, W. (1984). *Contraceptive Technology 1984–1985*. New York: Irvington Publications.

Hayes, K., Danks, D. M., and Gibas, H. (1972). Cytomegalovirus in human milk. *New England Journal of Medicine*, 287: 177–78.

Health Education Associates. (1984). *Why do mothers breast-feed?* Glenside, PA: Health Education Associates, Inc. Pamphlet.

Heartwell, S. F. and Schlesselman, S. (1983). Risk of uterine perforation among users of intrauterine devices. *Obstetrics and Gynecology,* 61(1): 31–36.

Hemmings, W. A. (1981). Maternal diet and colicky breastfed infants. Letter. *Lancet,* 2: 418–19.

Hide, D. W. and Guyer, B. M. (1985). Clinical manifestations of allergy related to breast- and cow's milk-feeding. *Pediatrics,* 76(6): 973–74.

Hinds, M. deC. (1982, March 12). FDA asks Wyeth to recall infant food short on vitamin. *New York Times,* A1, A14.

Hitchcock, N. E., Gracey, M., and Gilmour, A. I. (1985). The growth of breast fed and artificially fed infants from birth to twelve months. *Acta Paediatr. Scand.,* 74(2): 240–45.

Holborow, P. L. and Berry, P. (1982). Breast feeding and hyperactivity. (letter) *Medical Journal of Australia,* 1(2): 62.

Hormann, E. (1971). *Relactation: A Guide to Breastfeeding the Adopted Baby.* Belmont, MA.

Hunziker, U. A. and Barr, R. G. (1986). Increased carrying reduces infant crying: a randomized controlled trial. *Pediatrics,* 77(5): 641–48.

Jacobson, H. B. (1982). Breastmilk contaminants—an ill-defined risk. *The Lactation Review,* 6: 21–27, 35.

Jakobsson, I. and Lindberg, T. (1983). Cow's milk proteins cause infantile colic in breast-fed infants: A double-blind crossover study. *Pediatrics,* 71(2): 268–71.

Jelliffe, D. B. (1955). *Infant Nutrition in the Tropics and Subtropics.* Geneva: World Health Organization.

Jelliffe, D. B. (1968, February). Breast-milk and the world protein gap. *Clinical Pediatrics,* 7, 96–99.

Jelliffe, D. B. and Jelliffe, E. F. P. (1971). Human milk as an ecological force. Paper delivered before First Asian Nutritional Congress, Hyderabad, India.

Jelliffe, D. B. and Jelliffe, E. F. P., eds. (1971, August). The uniqueness of human milk. A symposium, *American Journal of Clinical Nutrition*, pp. 968–1024.

Jelliffe, D. B. and Jelliffe, E. F. P. (1983). Recent scientific knowledge concerning breastfeeding, *Rev. Epidem. et Sante Publ.*, 31: 367–73.

Jelliffe, D. B. and Jelliffe, E. F. P. (1984). Breast-milk policy. (1984). *World Health Forum*, 5: 37–38.

Jenkins, G. H. C. (1981). Milk-drinking mothers with colicky babies. *Lancet*, 2: 261.

Johnson, C. A. (1983). An evaluation of breast pumps currently available on the American market. *Clinical Pediatrics*, 22(1): 40–45.

Jones, J. B., Mehta, N. R., and Hamosh, M. (1982). a-Amylase in preterm human milk. *Journal of Pediatric Gastroenterology and Nutrition*, 1(1): 43–48.

Katcher, A. L. and Lanese, M. G. (1985). Breast-feeding by employed mothers: A reasonable accommodation in the work place. *Pediatrics*, 75(4): 644–47.

Kayner, C. E. and Zagar, J. A. (1983). Breast-feeding and sexual response. *Journal of Family Practice*, 17(1): 69–73.

Kendrick, E. (1980). Testing for environmental contaminants in breast milk. *Pediatrics*, 66: 470–72.

Kibrick, S. (1979). Herpes simplex virus in breast milk. *Pediatrics*, 64(3): 390–91.

Kinsey, A. C., Pomeroy, W. B., Martin, C. E., and Gebhart, P. H. (1953). *Sexual Behavior in the Human Female*. Philadelphia: Saunders.

Klaus, M. H. and Kennell, J. H. (1976). *Maternal-Infant Bonding*. St. Louis: C. V. Mosby.

Kon, S. K. and Cowie, A. T., eds. (1961). *Milk: The Mammary Gland and Its Secretion*, 2 vols. New York: Academic Press, Inc.

Kovar, M. G., Serdula, M. K., Marks, J. S., and Fraser, D. W. (1984). Review of the epidemiologic evidence for an association between infant feeding and infant health. *Supplement: Report on the Task Force on the Assessment of the Scientific Evidence Relating to Infant-Feeding Practices and Infant Health, Pediatrics*, 74(4, part 2): 615–38.

Kramer, M. S. (1981). Do breast-feeding and delayed introduction of solid foods protect against subsequent obesity? *Journal of Pediatrics*, 98(6): 833–37.

Kramer, M. S. and Moroz, B. (1981). Do breast-feeding and delayed introduction of solid foods protect against subsequent atopic eczema? *Journal of Pediatrics*, 98(4): 546–50.

Ladas, A. K. (1970). How to help mothers breastfeed: Deductions from a survey. *Clinical Pediatrics*, 9: 702–5.

La Leche League News, bimonthly newsletters, La Leche League International, Franklin Park, IL.

Lamb, M. E. (1982). Early contact and maternal-infant bonding: One decade later. *Pediatrics*, 70(5): 763–68.

Latham, M. C. (1985, August 20). Breast-feeding more important than contraceptives in population control. Talk given to 13th International Congress of Nutrition in Brighton, England.

L'Esperance, C. M. (1980). Pain or pleasure: The dilemma of early breastfeeding. *Birth and the Family Journal*, 7(1): 21–26.

Lindberg, T. and Skude, G. (1982). Amylase in human milk. *Pediatrics*, 70(2): 235–38.

Little, J. W., III (associate professor of plastic surgery at Georgetown University School of Medicine and director of the division of plastic and reconstructive surgery at the Georgetown University Medical Center). (1984, September 17). Personal communication.

Lothe, L., Lindberg, T., and Jakobsson, I. (1982). Cow's milk formula as a cause of infantile colic: A double-blind study. *Pediatrics*, 70(1): 7–10.

Lumpkin, M. D., Samson, W. K., and McCann, S. M. (1983). Hypothalamic and pituitary sites of action of oxytocin to alter prolactin secretion in the rat. *Endocrinology*, 112(5): 1711–17.

Lyon, A. J. (1983). Effects of smoking on breast feeding. *Archives of Diseases of Children*, 58(5): 378–80.

MacFarlane, A. (1975). Olfaction in the development of social preferences in the human neonate. *In Ciba Foundation Symposium 33 (new series)*, The human neonate in parent-infant interaction. Amsterdam: Associated Scientific Publishers.

MacMahon, B., Lin, T. M., Lowe, C. R, et al. (1970). Lactation and cancer of the breast. A summary of an international body. *Bulletin of the World Health Organization*, 42, 185–94.

Marano, H. (1979, March 5). The problem with protein. *New York*, 49–52.

Marano, H. (1979, October 29). Breast or bottle: New evidence in an old debate. *New York*, 56–60.

Marmet, C. (1981). Manual expression of breast milk: Marmet technique. Franklin Park, IL: La Leche League (Reprint No. 107).

Marmet, C. and Shell, E. (1984). *How to Solve Neonatal Sucking Problems: A Key to Overcoming Sore Nipples, Slower Gain and Failure to Thrive*. Los Angeles: Lactation Institute.

Marmet, C. and Shell, E. (1984). Training neonates to suck correctly, *Maternal & Child Nursing*, 9(6): 401–7.

Martinez, G. A. and Dodd, D. A. (1983). 1981 milk feeding patterns in the United States during the first 12 months of life. *Pediatrics*, 71(2): 166–170.

Martinez, G. A. and Kreiger, F. W. (1985). 1984 milk-feeding patterns in the United States. *Pediatrics*, 76(6): 1004–08.

Masters, W. H. and Johnson, V. E. (1966) *Human Sexual Response*. Boston: Little, Brown.

Matheny, R. and Picciano, M. F. (1986). Feeding and growth characteristics of human milk-fed infants. *Journal Am. Diet Assn.*, 86(3): 327–31.

Mauk, S. (1984, April). Children: Breast-feeding and work. *Working Woman*, pp. 43–44.

McKeith, R. (1969). Breast feed for the first two months. *Developmental Medicine and Child Neurology*, 11: 277–78.

Mehta, N. R., Jones, J. B., and Hamosh, M. (1982). Lipases in preterm human milk: Ontogeny and physiologic significance. *Journal of Pediatric Gastroenterology and Nutrition*, 1(3): 317–26.

Miller, S. A. and Chopra, J. G. (1984). Problems with human milk and infant formulas. *Supplement: Report on the Task Force on the Assessment of the Scientific Evidence Relating to Infant-Feeding Practices and Infant Health, Pediatrics*, 74(4, part 2): 639–47.

Montague, A. (1971). *Touching: The Human Significance of the Skin*. New York: Columbia University Press.

Moore, B. J. and Brasel, J. A. (1984). Nursing uses fat stored during pregnancy. *Journal of Nutrition*.

Moore, D. H., Charney, J. Kramarsky, B., Lasfargues, E. Y., Sarkar, N. H., Brennan, M. J., Burrows, J. H., Sirsat, S. M., Paymaster, J. C., and Vaidya, A. B. (1971). Search for a human breast cancer virus. *Nature*, 229: 611–14.

Naveh, Y., Hazani, A., and Berant, M. (1981). Copper deficiency with cow's milk diet. *Pediatrics*, 68(3): 397–99.

Neifert, M. R., Seacat, J. M., and Jobe, W. E. (1985). Lactation failure due to insufficient glandular development of the breast. *Pediatrics*, 76(5): 823–28.

Neville, M. C. and Neifert, M. R., eds. (1983). *Lactation: Physiology, Nutrition, and Breast-Feeding*. New York: Plenum Press.

New York Times. (1979, November 10). 300,000 cans of infant formula are recalled over fear of illness. *The New York Times*, 48.

Newton, M. (1970). Breast-feeding by adoptive mother. *Journal of American Medical Association*, 212: 11.

Newton, M. and Newton, N. (1962). The normal course and management of lactation. *Clinical Obstetrics and Gynecology*, 5: 44–63.

Newton, N. (1955). *Maternal Emotions*. New York: Paul B. Hoeber, Inc. (Harper & Row.).

Newton, N. (1971, February 5). Interrelationship between various aspects of the female reproductive role: A review. Paper presented to annual meeting of American Psychopathological Association, New York.

Newton, N. and Newton, M. (1967). Psychologic aspects of lactation. *New England Journal of Medicine*, 277: 1179–88.

Newton, N. and Theotokatos, M. (1979). Breast-feeding during pregnancy in 503 women: Does a psychological weaning mechanism exist in humans?, in: *Proceedings of the 5th International Congress Psychosomatic Obstetrics & Gynecology* (Carenza, L. and Zichella, L., eds.). London: Academic Press, pp. 845–49.

Newton, N., Peeler, D., and Rawlins, C. (1968). Effect of lactation on maternal behavior in mice with comparative data on humans. *Lying-In: The Journal of Reproductive Medicine*, 1: 257–62.

Noone, R. B. (clinical associate professor of surgery of the University of Pennsylvania Medical School and director of the division of plastic surgery at Bryn Mawr Hospital). (1984, September 17). Personal communication.

O'Connor, M. E., Livingstone, D. S., Hannah, J., and Wilkins, D. (1983). Vitamin K deficiency and breast-feeding. *American Journal of Diseases of Children*, 137: 601–02.

Ojofeitimi, E. O. (1982). Effect of duration and frequency of breast-feeding on postpartum amenorrhea. *Pediatrics*, 69(2): 164–68.

Olds, S. W. (1985). *The Eternal Garden: Seasons of Our Sexuality*. New York: Times Books.

Olds, S. W. (1986). *The Working Parents Survival Guide*. New York: Bantam Books.

Olds, S. W. (1973, April). In praise of breastfeeding. *Ms.*, 10–14.

Olds, S. W. (1976, March). Breast-feeding is nature's way of saying mother knows best. *Today's Health*, 47–49.

Olds, S. W. (1977, September). Make breastfeeding a turn-on for you, a boon for your baby. *Be Alive*, 68–72.

Olds, S. W. (1980, January). All about breast-feeding: 25 vital questions and answers. *Parents*, 47–50.

Ory, H. W., Forrest, J. D., and Lincoln, R. (1983). *Making Choices: Evaluating the Health Risks and Benefits of Birth Control Methods*. New York: Alan Guttmacher Institute.

Orzalesi, M. (1982). Do breast and bottle fed babies require vitamin supplements? *Acta Paediatr. Scand. Suppl.* 299: 77.

Oski, F. A. (1980, January 17). Nutritional needs of infancy. The kindness of human milk. *Ethel and Jack Hausman Lectureship in Pediatrics*, North Shore University Hospital, Manhasset, New York.

Ostler, C. W. (1979). Initial feeding time of newborn infants: Effect upon first meconium passage and serum indirect bilirubin levels. *Health Care of Women*, 1(6): 2.

Page, H. J. and Lesthaeghe, R., eds. (1981). *Child-Spacing in Tropical Africa: Traditions and Change*. London: Academic Press.

Paine, R. and Coble, R. J. (1982). Breast-feeding and infant health in a rural U.S. community. *Am. J. Dis. Child.* 136, 36–38.

Papalia, D. E. and Olds, S. W. (1986). *Human Development*. New York: McGraw-Hill.

Papalia, D. E. and Olds, S. W. (1987). *A Child's World (4th Edition)*. New York: McGraw-Hill.

Parents Forum: How and at what ages have you weaned your children? (1982, July–Aug.). *Practical Parenting*, 8–9.

Parmalee, A. H., Wenner, W. H., and Schulz, H. R. (1964). Infant sleep patterns: From birth to 16 weeks of age. *Journal of Pediatrics*, 65: 576.

Paxson, C. L. and Cress, C. C. (1979). Survival of human milk leukocytes. *Journal of Pediatrics*, 94: 61.

Pearson, J. (1985, spring). A weaning. *Nurturing*, 90–91.

Peters, T., Golding, J., and Butler, N. R. (1985, January 5). Breast-feeding and childhood eczema. (letter) *Lancet*, 49–50.

Petschek, M. A. and Barber-Madden, R. (1984). Promoting prenatal care and breastfeeding in the workplace: The role of the occupational health nurse. Paper presented at the Greater New York Occupational Health Nurses Assn., Continuing Education Seminar, New York City, April 17.

Population Information Program (Johns Hopkins University). (1981, November–December). Breast-feeding, fertility, and family planning. *Population Reports*, Series J., no. 24, J525–J575.

Raiha, N. C. (1985). Nutritional proteins in milk and the protein requirement of normal infants. *Supplement: Current Issues in Feeding the Normal Infant, Pediatrics*, 75(1, part 2): 136–41.

Randall, Goldblum, Johnson, Garza, Nichols, Harris, and Goldman. (1981). Human milk banking I: Effect of container on immunological factors in mature milk. *Nutrition Research*, 1, 449–59.

Raphael, D. (1983, summer). Nursing the adopted baby. *Childbirth Educator*, 43–44.

Raphael, D. (1973). *The Tender Gift: Breastfeeding*. New York: Schocken Books.

Raphael, D. and Davis, F. (1985). *Only Mothers Know*. Westport, CT: Greenwood Press.

Reid, B., Smith, M., and Friedman, Z. (1980). Prostaglandins in human milk. *Pediatrics*, 66(8): 870–72.

Reynolds, D. W., Stagno, S., Hosty, T. S., Tiller, M., and Alford, C. A. (1973). Maternal cytomegalovirus excretion and perinatal infection. *New England Journal of Medicine*, 289(1): 1–5.

Riordan, J. and Riordan, M. (1984). Drugs in breast milk. *American Journal of Nursing*, 84(3): 328–32.

Robson, K. S. and Moss, H. A. (1970). Patterns and determinants of maternal attachment. *Journal of Pediatrics*, 77(6): 976–85.

Roepke, J. B. (1985, July 17). Losing weight while breastfeeding. Presentation at tenth international conference, La Leche League, Washington, DC.

Rogan, W. J., Bagniewska, A., and Damstra, T. (1980). Pollutants in breast milk. *New England Journal of Medicine*, 302: 1450–53.

Roseman, B. D. (1981). Sunkissed urine. Letter. *Pediatrics*, 67(3): 443.

Rossi, A. S. (1971, February). Maternalism, sexuality and the new feminism. Paper presented to annual meeting of American Psychopathological Association, New York City.

Russell, M. (1976). Human olfactory communication. *Nature*, 260: 520–22.

Rutishauser, I. H., McKay, H. M., and Wahlqvist, M. L. (1982). Does breast feeding have nutritional advantages over bottle feeding? *Australian Family Physician*, 11(4): 249–53.

Scanlon, J. W. (1976, February 19). Effects of local anesthetics administered to parturient women on the neurological and behavorial performance of newborn children. *Bulletin of New York Academy of Medicine*, 2: 231.

Schaefer, O. (1969). Cancer of the breast and lactation. *Canadian Medical Association Journal*, 100: 625–26.

Scherz, R. G. (1980). Premie nipples: A potential aspiration hazard. *Pediatrics*, 65(1): 163–4.

Schmeck, H. M., Jr. (1985, August 10). Brain hormone regulating fertility is discovered. *New York Times*, 5.

Scientific American. (1981). Science and the citizen. *Scientific American*, 245(2): 68.

Shenon, P. (1985, September 24). Agencies split in baby-formula case. *New York Times*, A28.

Shinwell, E. D. and Gorodischer, R. (1982). Totally vegetarian diets and infant nutrition. *Pediatrics*, 70(4): 582–86.

Short, R. V. (1984). Breast feeding. *Scientific American*, 250(4): 35–41.

Shostak, M. (1981). *Nisa: The Life and Words of a !Kung Woman*. Cambridge, MA: Harvard University Press.

Shull, M. W., Reed, R. B., Valadian, I., Palombo, R., Thorne, H., and Dwyer, J. T. (1977). Velocities of growth in vegetarian preschool children. *Pediatrics*, 60: 410–17.

Slaven, S. and Harvey, D. (1981). Unlimited suckling time improves breast feeding. *Lancet*, 1: 392–93.

Solomon, S. (1981, December 6). The controversy over infant formula. *The New York Times Magazine*, 92 + .

Specker, B., Tsang, R. C., and Hollis, B. Effect of race and maternal diet on breast milk vitamin D and 25-hydroxyvitamin D concentrations. *American Journal of Diseases of Children*.

Spock, B. and Rothenberg, M. B. (1985). *Dr. Spock's Baby and Child Care*. New York: Pocket Books.

Stewart, D. (1979). *Fathering and Career: A Healthy Balance*. Seattle: the pennypress.

Straub, W. J. (1960). Malfunction of the tongue. Part I: The abnormal swallowing habit: Its cause, effects and results in relation to orthodontic treatment and speech therapy. *American Journal of Orthodontics*, 46: 404–24.

Sullivan-Bolyai, J. Z., Fife, K. H., Jacobs, R. F., Miller, Z., and Corey, L. (1983). Disseminated neonatal herpes simplex virus type 1 from a maternal breast lesion. *Pediatrics*, 71(3): 455–57.

Sulman, F. G. (1970). *Hypothalamic Control of Lactation*. Heidelberg: Springer-Verlag.

SUNY-Buffalo. (1983, spring). Viruses/breast milk. *SUNY-Buffalo*, 12.

Thoman, E. B., Connor, R. L., and Levine, S. (1970). Lactation suppresses adrenal corticosteroid activity and aggressiveness in rats. *Journal of Comparative and Physiological Psychology*, 70: 364–69.

Thoman, E. B., Wetzel, A., and Levine, S. (1968). Lactation prevents disruption of temperature regulation and suppresses adrenocortical activity in rats. *Communications in Behavioral Biology*, Part A, 2, 165–71, Abstract No. 10680066.

Thomsen, A. C., Espersen, T., and Maigaard, S. (1984). Course and treatment of milk stasis, noninfectious inflammation of the breast, and infectious mastitis in nursing women. *American Journal of Obstetrics and Gynecology*, 149: 492–95.

Vuorenkoski, V., et al. (1969). The effect of cry stimulus on the temperature of the lactating breast of primipara. A thermographic study. *Experientia*, 25: 1286–7.

Waletzky, L. R., M.D. (1979). Husbands' problems with breast-feeding. *American Journal of Orthopsychiatry*, 49(2): 349–52.

Waller, H. (1957). *The Breasts and Breast Feeding*. London: William Heinemann.

Weichert, C. E. (1979). Lactational reflex recovery in breast-feeding failure. *Pediatrics*, 63(5): 799–803.

White, G. J. and White, M. (1984). Breastfeeding and drugs in human milk. *Veterinary and Human Toxicology*, 26, Supplement 1, 1–26.

Whitehead, R. G. (1985). Infant physiology, nutritional requirements, and lactational adequacy. *American Journal of Clinical Nutrition*, 41, 447–58.

Whitfield, M. (1981). Validity of routine clinical test weighing as a measure of the intake of breast-fed infants. *Archives of Diseases of Children*, 56: 91.

Whitley, N. N. (1970). Breast feeding the premature. *American Journal of Nursing*, 70: 1909.

Wickizer, T. M. and Brilliant, L. B. (1981). Testing for polychlorinated biphenyls in human milk. *Pediatrics*, 68: 411–15.

Williams, H. H. (1961). Differences between cow's and human milk. *Journal of the American Medical Association*, 175: 104–7.

Winick, M. (1985, February). Breastfeeding: The more we learn, the better it is. *American Baby*, pp. 63, 76.

Winters, R. W. (1981, May 26). The therapeutic role of human milk in feeding premature infants. Presentation to National Association of Science Writers, Rockefeller University, New York.

Young, H. B., Buckley, A. E., Hamza, B., and Mandarano, C. (1982). Milk and lactation: Some social and developmental correlates among 1,000 infants. *Pediatrics*, 69(2): 169–75.

Recommended Readings

Brazelton, T. Berry, M.D. (1985). *Working and Caring*. Reading, Mass.: Merloyd Lawrence Books (Addison-Wesley). A compassionate, understanding book by a noted pediatrician that focuses on three families: a professional couple, a working-class couple, and a single mother. Good advice on many of the issues faced by working parents, including managing breastfeeding around a work schedule.

Brewster, Dorothy P. (1979). *You Can Breastfeed Your Baby . . . even in special situations*. Emmaus, PA: Rodale Press. Written for mothers and babies with special problems, such as medical conditions of either one, certain physical handicaps, and various other situations, this book is informative, warm, and encouraging.

Brody, Jane, (1982). *Jane Brody's Nutrition Book*. New York: Bantam. A comprehensive, sensible guide to good, healthy eating, with special suggestions for pregnant and nursing women, vegetarians, and children.

Bumgarner, Norma Jane. (1982). *Mothering Your Nursing Toddler*. Franklin Park, IL: La Leche League International, Inc. This book helps mothers who are breastfeeding older children manage in a practice that is common in other parts of the world but is generally unpopular in the United States. Written with humor and warmth, it provides suggestions for getting enough rest, avoiding embarrassment in public, and weaning a nurser who is reluctant.

Eisenberg, Arlene, Heidi E. Murkoff, and Sandee E. Hathaway. (1986). *What to Eat When You're Expecting.* New York: Workman. A medically accurate, easy-to-follow guide to good, nutritious eating during pregnancy and lactation, with a bonus of 100 specially created recipes.

Eisenberg, Arlene, Heidi E. Murkoff, and Sandee E. Hathaway. (1984). *What to Expect When You're Expecting.* New York: Workman. An excellent, comprehensive description of pregnancy, month to month, that incorporates the most up-to-date research on care for both mother and baby.

Goldfarb, Johanna and Edith Tibbetts. (1980). *Breastfeeding Handbook: A Practical Reference for Physicians, Nurses and Other Health Professionals.* Hillside, NJ: Enslow. This well-organized, well-referenced manual provides background information along with practical suggestions for professionals.

Grams, Marilyn, M.D. (1985). *Breastfeeding Success for Working Mothers.* Sheridan, WY: Achievement Press. Written by a physician who breastfed two babies while pursuing her career, this book presents her innovative solutions in a chatty, personal way.

La Leche League International. (1983). *The Womanly Art of Breastfeeding.* Third edition. New York: New American Library. This revised version of the first book to have appeared on the topic has many practical suggestions and represents the philosophy of this organization, which has done so much to help nursing mothers.

Lappe, Frances Moore. (1975). *Diet for a Small Planet.* New York: Ballantine. The book that created a mini-revolution in American kitchens by showing cooks how to combine non-meat foods in the proper proportions to produce high-grade protein nutrition that is equivalent to, or better than, meat proteins—and is economical, besides.

Lawrence, Ruth A. (1985). *Breastfeeding: A Guide for the Medi-

cal Profession. Second edition. St. Louis: Mosby. A manual for physicians, nurses, and other health-care professionals, drawing on up-to-date research to help professionals as they help nursing mothers.

Lesko, Wendy and Matthew. (1985). *The Maternity Sourcebook*. New York: Warner Books. A big, readable, up-to-date, information-packed guide for expectant and new parents that offers help on what to do and directions on where to go for more specific help on a variety of issues, such as health insurance, first-aid techniques, and many other common parental concerns.

Neville, Margaret C. and Marianne R. Neifert, Editors. (1983). *Lactation: Physiology, Nutrition, and Breast-Feeding*. New York: Plenum Press. A thorough, up-to-date professional reference book containing articles by 18 contributors who cover the history of breastfeeding, its physiology, management of both typical and special situations, and a number of controversial issues.

Olds, Sally Wendkos. (1985). *The Eternal Garden: Seasons of Our Sexuality*. New York: Times Books. A description of sexual development throughout life, illustrated by personal accounts from individuals ranging in age from 20 to 83 concerning significant turning points in their own lives, which are then interpreted in the light of both classic and contemporary research. In-depth exploration of the impact of pregnancy, breastfeeding, and child rearing on sexual relationships.

Olds, Sally Wendkos. (1983). *The Working Parents Survival Guide*. New York: Bantam Books. An in-depth manual full of practical tips for such issues as finding and evaluating good child care, saving time and energy in running a home, creating alternative work schedules, and the special concerns of both married and single parents.

Papalia, Diane and Sally Wendkos Olds. (1987). *A Child's World. Fourth edition*. New York: McGraw-Hill. An easy-to-read summary of the most up-to-date information about child development, from conception through adolescence, with many suggestions for practical application of research findings. This book is widely used as a college text and an accompaniment to a video course, but it can also be read independently.

Parkes, Alan, S. (1976). *Patterns of Sexuality and Reproduction*. London: Oxford University Press. This interesting book contains some intriguing accounts of different cultural efforts to increase the yield of milk, plus some records of individual women's milk production.

Pryor, Karen. (1973). *Nursing Your Baby*. New York: Pocket Books. One of the first books on breastfeeding to appear, this work by a behavioral psychologist draws on scientific research to help breastfeeding mothers.

Raphael, Dana. (1970). *Breastfeeding: The Tender Gift*. New York: Schocken. An anthropologist's look at breastfeeding, with special emphasis on the role of the "doula," the person who mothers the mother, and suggestions for finding and working with one.

Raphael, Dana and Flora Davis. (1985). *Only Mothers Know*. Westport, CT: Greenwood Press. An anthropological account of the ways in which women in various countries feed their babies, in response to complex social and economic forces.

Riordan, Jan. (1983). *A Practical Guide to Breastfeeding*. St. Louis: Mosby. A comprehensive professional reference, especially geared toward giving practicing nurses the information they need to help breastfeeding mothers.

Robertson, Laurel, Carol Flinders, and Bronwen Godrey. (1976). *Laurel's Kitchen: A Handbook for Vegetarian Cookery and Nutrition*. New York: Bantam. A classic for vegetarian gourmets, this book presents a philosophy of vegetarianism and many recipes.

Spock, Benjamin and Michael B. Rothenberg. (1985). *Dr. Spock's Baby and Child Care*. New York: Pocket Books. This new, extensively revised version of the classic child care book is a compendium of valuable information. Its section on breastfeeding is much expanded from previous editions, and more helpful and encouraging.

Index

A Note to Our Readers

Were there questions about your own breastfeeding experience that were not answered in the pages of this book? Or did you learn things from your own personal or professional experience that could help other nursing families? If you have any questions or comments at all, we would very much like to hear from you. We'll try to be as helpful as possible to you, and we'll also keep this information in mind for possible inclusion in our next revision. (Some of the new information in this edition of *The Complete Book of Breastfeeding* was inspired by just such letters from readers of the first edition.)

Just write to either Sally Wendkos Olds or Marvin S. Eiger, M.D., c/o Bantam Books, Inc., 666 Fifth Avenue, New York, NY 10103.